"What a timely book this is. The world is getting angrier, and for many, the skills needed to work with this emotion are sadly lacking. This practical book offers information and tools to guide women with their unexpressed and destructively expressed anger. When women can use their anger in service of life, health, and the world—we will see a beautiful transformation. This book is a gift for women, men, and the world."

> —**Ann Bradney**, founder and director of the Radical Aliveness Institute, who runs a three-year program for Peace Leadership in Israel and Palestine

"This is a thoughtful approach that zeroes in on possibility rather than punishment. Although 'to release' can mean to momentarily reconnect with, I promise you it is in a constructive and empowering way. Karyne Wilner delivers with all of her best insight, steeped in decades of both clinical and heartfelt, no-nonsense practice."

> —**Jo Standing**, one/we; author; and corporate and military wellness facilitator

"Karyne Wilner has been on the forefront of the somatic psychotherapy movement for many decades. *Releasing Toxic Anger for Women* is a culmination of her work. In this book, Karyne Wilner synthesizes an extensive body of knowledge on an embodied approach to working with women and anger. Here you will discover a rich panoply of exercises, insights, and creative approaches for women to reclaim the positive aspects of human anger."

> —**Brian Gleason, LCSW, CCEP**, practicing psychotherapist, teacher, writer, cofounder of The Center for Exceptional Marriage, and author of *Mortal Spirit* and *Relative to Everything*

"Karyne Wilner provides an excellent explanation of the important influence of toxic anger on women's health, and provides real-life strategies to ameliorate it."

> —**Justin P. Lavin Jr., MD, FACOG**, professor and chairman emeritus in the department of obstetrics and gynecology at Cleveland Clinic Akron General

"Karyne Wilner masterfully presents the best and most time-tested, state-of-the-art solutions for both understanding and overcoming anger, along with all of the psychological, physical, and spiritual toxicity it can cause. She speaks to her readers as both a woman with a story to tell, and a psychologist with many decades of experience helping countless women to massively improve their lives by using her highly effective strategies."

> —**Michael S. Broder, PhD**, psychologist, author, and trainer of mental health professionals—whose books include *Helping Adults to Grow Up* and *Seven Steps to Your Best Life*

T0262496

"As a psychotherapist with decades of experience, Karyne Wilner has written a much-needed book that dispels negative beliefs held about women and anger. She dismisses the guilt and shame bound in those beliefs and in its place, imbued with insight and wisdom, provides the reader with a practical guide through which to identify, understand, and heal what Wilner has termed as 'toxic anger.' It is an educational and liberating read!"

—**Laurie Keene**, dean of the Barbara Brennan School of Healing,
therapist, and author of *Awakening to The Truth of Who You Are*

"Drawing on professional and personal experiences, Karyne Willner beautifully illuminates the impact of the mind–body connection to the poison of anger through her book, *Releasing Toxic Anger for Women*. This book is a powerful and unique tool of deep expertise on how to move beyond the physical and mental impacts of anger on the body. A brilliant must-read for all women in need of self-healing work."

—**Bindu Babu, MD, PhD**, founder and president of Hearts of Change;
and author of *My Soulmate, My Love, My Narcissist*

"*Releasing Toxic Anger for Women* is a powerful resource for women who want to have fulfilling relationships where they can be assertive. Karyne Wilner masterfully teaches us with simple, practical tools how to identify anger, discover its original source, and how to release and transform it. Wilner's somatic focus will teach psychotherapists how to get results with clients of any gender. I'm thrilled to have this resource for my students."

—**Kate Holt, RN, ACCEP**, in private practice helping people live
more satisfying lives, and trains and supervises Core Energetics Practitioners
internationally

"Karyne Wilner writes, 'Anger doesn't knock on the door and announce itself,' and so she has presented us the opportunity to be prepared in how we greet it when it does come! This book maps out an exceptionally rich journey allowing readers the chance to explore and experience the deepest wisdom of somatic expression, and to move from reaction into self-awareness and presence. It is accessible, practical, and incredibly thorough."

—**Aylee Welch, LICSW**, founder and director of Seattle School of
Body-Psychotherapy, and longtime social worker and activist

"This is such an empowering book for women! Karyne Wilner brings awareness to the physical symptoms and chronic illnesses resulting from suppressed anger. She identifies a full range of states of anger suppression and behaviors, along with clearly set out exercises to facilitate a deep and integrated healing. I highly recommend this book for any women who want to transform their anger and live a life of positivity and vitality."

—**Andrea Alexander**, founder and director of the Institute of
Body Psychotherapy in Australia

RELEASING

Somatic Practices & CBT Skills to

TOXIC

Transform Negative Thoughts,

ANGER

Soothe Stress & Stay True to Yourself

for WOMEN

KARYNE B. WILNER, PSYD

New Harbinger Publications, Inc.

Publisher's Note

This publication is designed to provide accurate and authoritative information in regard to the subject matter covered. It is sold with the understanding that the publisher is not engaged in rendering psychological, financial, legal, or other professional services. If expert assistance or counseling is needed, the services of a competent professional should be sought.

NEW HARBINGER PUBLICATIONS is a registered trademark of New Harbinger Publications, Inc.

New Harbinger Publications is an employee-owned company.

Copyright © 2024 by Karyne B. Wilner
New Harbinger Publications, Inc.
5720 Shattuck Avenue
Oakland, CA 94609
www.newharbinger.com

Cover design by Amy Shoup

Acquired by Elizabeth Hollis Hansen

Edited by Kandace Little

Library of Congress Cataloging-in-Publication Data on file

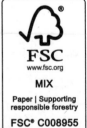

Printed in the United States of America

26   25   24

10   9   8   7   6   5   4   3   2   1   First Printing

To my parents

Stanley D. Miller and Evelyn Wilner Miller.

Thank you for supporting my dreams

and my goals.

To my mentor

John C. Pierrakos, MD.

Thank you for teaching me how to open my heart

and love.

To my friend and colleague

Irene Bryan, PhD.

You left too soon. I wasn't ready to say goodbye.

Contents

Foreword

So many times, I've walked out of a meeting with a colleague or left a conversation with a friend only to have her say, "I was so damn pissed off! I can't believe how angry I am!" Having heard her say nothing during the meeting to indicate her anger, I'd ask, "So why didn't you say something?" The reply would always be some form of "I didn't want to come off as rude," or "I didn't want be that angry woman," or "What was I going to do?" On the other hand, under similar circumstances, a different woman would rip into the other person, lashing out with a surprising level of anger that seemed unwarranted given the situation.

When it comes to feeling, acknowledging, and expressing anger, sentiment can range from denial to passivity to helplessness and victimhood to blind rage and outward aggression. As a long-term pattern, such extremes are physically, emotionally, and spiritually unhealthy for women. They negate the possibility of constructive engagement that opens dialogue, sets appropriate boundaries, and improves relationships.

Whatever your tendency with anger, Dr. Karyne B. Wilner's new book, *Releasing Toxic Anger for Women: Somatic Practices and CBT Skills to Transform Negative Thoughts, Soothe Stress, and Stay True to Yourself,* holds important teaching for you. You will learn to feel and own your anger, no longer numb to your feelings, blind to anger's source, or unconsciously attracting it. The strategies, tools and techniques she provides will, with practice, enable you to deal with your anger in ways that will surprise and delight you. In the process, your health and sense of well-being will improve, and the quality of every important relationship will be enhanced.

The approach Dr. Wilner has honed is backed by sound scientific research. Each chapter is filled with stories about real people. Since the patterns she identifies are common to humanity, don't be surprised when you recognize yourself, a good friend, or a colleague. In fact, expect to see your habituated ways of denying, avoiding, exacerbating, or antagonizing, or whatever your preferred approach to anger happens to be.

When she offers a practice, experiment with it…and stay with it. Be it journaling, breathing and awareness exercises, physical movement and postures, meditations, or more, they are all tried and true, and they all work, so practice, practice, practice. You're sure to find a favorite technique or two. Just know that the more you commit and follow through, the more natural your favorite practice will feel as you learn to move with greater conscious awareness and to experience more deeply what's happening within your mind, body, emotions, and spirit.

Sometimes the transformation of anger from held and unexpressed to boiling over—and then to a sense of clarity, a feeling of relief, the presence of peace—happens almost instantly. And, most often, it happens over time. Whatever your experience, stay the course. I promise you: these tools and techniques work. I speak with certainty because Dr. Wilner taught them to me a few decades ago. I've used them ever since because of their power to transform anger, whether frozen and cold or steamy hot, into the peace and calm I enjoy today. *Releasing Toxic Anger for Women* can do the same for you too.

Enjoy your journey from anger to greater self-awareness, peace, and love, all through deliberate movement and enhanced consciousness.

—Teressa Moore Griffin
Principal, Spirit of Purpose, LLC
Institute of Core Energetics, Board Chair

Acknowledgments

I give special thanks to John C. Pierrakos, in memoriam, my mentor and teacher who introduced me to body psychotherapy and helped me understand the interconnection between the body, anger, and health. My dissertation's hypothesis that anger management, using CBT, and bodymind techniques would help decrease blood pressure levels led to the concepts and exercises embedded in this book. I want to thank the subjects of my research and the medical center staff at the Philadelphia College of Osteopathic Medicine, whose participation in data collection added reliability and validity to the results.

I have gratitude for my parents, Evelyn Wilner Miller and Stanley D. Miller, who unintentionally taught me about the interaction between anger, loss, and health. In living their shared experiences and observing their health struggles, I learned in vivo about the impact of emotion, suppressed and expressed, on the body.

I am grateful to Ray Birdwhistell, now deceased, my dissertation advisor at the University of Pennsylvania who ignited my interest in nonverbal communications and all things to do with the body.

I give thanks to my husband, Jack Irwin, who passed away in 2015, and my daughter, Nicole Wilner, who both recognized the importance of my research and time involvement, even when it meant that I would be with them less. Finally, I appreciate the gentle prodding of Irvin Jennings, my life partner, who helped me get this project out of a file cabinet and off the ground, and whose thoughts about women's anger have been insightful.

Special thanks to my illustrator, Eric Lavin, for his sensitive depiction of somatic practices; to my first reader, Sarah E. Brown; and to the editors at New Harbinger for their understanding of my goals and help in getting my message across.

INTRODUCTION

Anger Hurts Your Health

You may be aware that you are angry. Or, like me, you may be unaware of the vast amount of anger you carry in your body. Either way, anger has a negative effect. Anger, whether expressed or repressed, has the power to wreck homes and relationships. Arguments can be physical and loud or avoided altogether: couples and families scream at each other or get completely quiet, shutting down communication for days.

Society-at-large perceives anger as dangerous and expects people, but especially women, to repress it. Women who show their anger are seen as mean or out of control, and little girls grow up learning that expressing anger is wrong. However, repressing anger may set the stage for serious health issues in the future. Because of these teachings, angry feelings remain tamped down in your body, in an out-of-awareness state, causing hormones to release that create a toxic environment within. The hormones cortisol, adrenaline, epinephrine, and noradrenaline upset the natural state of your organs and set the stage for an aggressive expression of anger, anger suppression, stress, illness, and disease (Christensen and Smith 1993; Everson et al. 1998; Julkunen, Idanpaan-Heikkila, and Saaeinen 1993; Lahad et al. 1997). Even fetuses feel the effect of anger. When parents-to-be argue and fight, the disparate sounds cause small bodies to contract in the womb. In fact, research ties physical and mental health issues that occur later in life to prenatal stress (Lange 2011; Meany 2018; Stern 1990; Wilner 2020).

Because you are not the superwomen you imagine yourself to be, you, like many other women, may make life difficult for yourself. Setting the bar of achievement too high, you may struggle with issues around work, parenting, running a household, and caring for others. In the mix, you stop caring for yourself, and you get angry. Current events may motivate you to fight for equality and socioeconomic change. But along with many of us, you are thwarted when you hit your head against the proverbial brick wall and glass ceiling. Then you get stuck in patterns of anger that lead to your own internal suffering.

The intention of this seven-step program is to help you deal with these struggles in healthy ways. This book teaches you to become aware of your anger and to change its form, so that it can move from something dark, ugly, and unhealthy to a compassionate expression of a higher purpose and love.

A Body-Based Approach

I once received a call from a former ballerina. She had danced professionally until one of the directors molested her. Suppressing her anger in response to the trauma, she developed a phobia to anything related to dance. Yet she still loved the profession and wanted to conquer her fear. When I asked her why she called me for help, the answer was that she had been looking for a body therapist. Whether or not you are a dancer or an athlete, you may be attracted to body therapies and holistic health, attend yoga classes regularly, go for acupuncture, sign up for reiki, massage, or craniosacral work, and perhaps even visit integrative medicine practitioners and naturopaths. You may bring your children to the gym with you, not wanting to miss a workout session, and you could appear to be more health oriented than your partner, taking responsibility for scheduling doctor's appointments for both of you.

As interested as you may be in body-oriented things, you want more knowledge and skills concerning anger: how to identify it, communicate it, and use it for problem solving and relationship enhancement. Trying to be nice or kind all the time reveals a desire to mask negative emotions and at the same time feeds the notion that the expression of reasonable anger is wrong. If you smile and appear upbeat even when the situation is unpleasant, you are failing to establish sound boundaries with abusive and untrustworthy people. You may do this out of fear of being accused of lacking compassion, or worse, of being called a "witch" or a "bitch."

Eventually anger causes you to explode either outwardly toward others or inwardly, toward yourself. You experience injustice, feel misunderstood, and react to rejection, saying, "After all I have done for you." You become aroused as stress hormones laced with cortisol and adrenaline flow into your bloodstream. Then, you may lose your temper, screaming and throwing things, and develop a reputation for being of unsound mind or the victim of fluctuating hormones. Or you turn your anger inward, and your body pays the price. These same chemicals invade your bloodstream and have the potential to cause harm later in life. Heart disease, the number one killer in the United States, is particularly problematic for women because it is often misdiagnosed due to the medical field's belief that it is more prevalent in men (Harburg et al. 2003; Knox and Follman 1993; Lai and Linden 1992; Lawler et al. 1993; Lawler, Wilcox, and Anderson 1995; Maas and Appelman 2010; Martin, Gordon, and Lounsbury 1998; Suarez et al. 1998; Vögele, Jarvis, and Cheeseman 1997).

Suppressed anger has also been associated with cancer, the second leading cause of death after heart disease in the United States and the primary cause of death for women between the ages of thirty and fifty-four (OWH 2023). Standardized tests found that women diagnosed with cancer had unnaturally low anger scores, providing strong evidence that women were suppressing their anger and putting their health at risk (Guidi et al. 2021; Linkins and Comstock 1990; Morris et al. 1981; Zonderman, Costa, and McCrae 1989). Additionally, anger results after a cancer diagnosis because now we're faced with uncomfortable and painful treatments, changed plans, pain, disfigurement, and a loss of control over our lives (Turk, Meichenbaum, and Genest 1983).

In the last fifty years, cases involving other illnesses, especially immune disorders, have skyrocketed. Genetics can't entirely be at the root of the problem—genes don't change that fast. More likely, stress, an unfriendly combination of fear and anger that takes up residence in our bodies, plays a role (Banafa, Suominen, and Sipila 2023; Boyle, Church II, and Byrnes 2005; Chaudhury and Banerjee 2020; Lehrer 2006; Rimes et al. 2016; Rodriguez 2012; Smyth et al. 2014; Truglia et al. 2006; Young 1992; Whitehead 1992). Autoimmune disease attacks three to four times more women than men, suggesting that women in today's world are carrying an unusual amount of tension, stress, and anger (Maté and Maté 2023; Selye 1978). According to behavioral health studies, we can best protect our health and respond to stress by tactfully, reasonably, and rationally verbalizing and communicating anger and by moving our bodies by engaging in exercise or dance (Ayakody, Gunadasa, and Hosker 2014; Capon et al. 2021; Chekroud et al. 2018; Dubbert 1992; Huddleston 1992; Singh et al. 2023; Wilner 1999; Young 1992; Zschucke, Gaudlitz, and Ströhle 2013).

The body-based exercises and techniques included in this book emphasize prevention and improving health. They are designed to help you tap into your body's knowledge, release past hurts, achieve forgiveness, and change your life for the better.

How Anger Showed Up in My Life

Growing up, I watched my parents' anger play out in front of me. Their anger marred the landscape of my childhood mostly because they never discussed it. Sparks would fly seemingly out of nowhere, then disappear. They shared common values, a love of reading, and a strong work ethic, but when it came to anger, they expressed it differently. Hers was overt and in your face; his was suppressed.

Mother's anger could be unpredictable and even vicious. I remember a look that could kill. Those eyes made me feel like the worst person in the world. What crime did I commit to draw such a response? Upset, I would run down the stairs to the basement and sit on a shelf in an unused coal cellar, brooding and secretly hating her. Even now as I write this, I think about the difficulty she had trusting others, expecting her best friends—bridge party ladies and close neighbors—to turn on her. For her, thoughts of betrayal were pervasive.

Dad's anger, on the other hand, was quiet and passive. His pleasant face and shy smile hid deeper feelings. He suppressed his anger, directing it toward me only when I did something he considered stupid like dropping a bowling ball into the outer lane during a competition—triggering a look laced with disgust. In response to my mother's anger, he left the house, shutting the door solidly behind him and going for a long walk. When I thought he was being unfairly attacked, I took his side to protect him, which, of course, often made things worse. Unfortunately, stress found an outlet in his physical body. He developed a number of digestive issues. A line from a poem I wrote describing him according to a childhood memory reads: "Fingers scratching naked, long legs; Opening up sores oozing blood."

Later, both my parents experienced major health events. At the time, I didn't have the knowledge to connect their health issues with chronic anger from stress, unresolved grief, and fear. But their ancestral trauma, personal losses, and frustrated ambitions affected their lives and the illnesses that led to their deaths.

Growing up, I was unaware of the repercussions unprocessed anger has on the body, but later, as I thought about my parents' health struggles, my gut instinct told me that a relationship exists between emotions and illness. I came to believe that if people were given the opportunity to deal with their feelings openly and honestly, they would have better outcomes. Influenced by my parents' inability to talk about difficult topics, I earned a master's degree in nonverbal communications; I studied with Ray Birdwhistell, a well-known anthropologist, at the University of Pennsylvania, where I learned healthy and helpful ways to deal with intense feelings and stressful situations.

A psychologist friend encouraged me to attend a seminar featuring the psychiatrist John C. Pierrakos, who cofounded Bioenergetics and developed Core Energetics, two well-known body therapies. As soon as I watched him give a demonstration session, I knew that I wanted to study with him; his understanding of the relationship between the mind, emotions, and the physical body corresponded exactly with my area of interest. The four-year training in Core Energetics, which I began in 1983, led to my immersion in the field of body psychotherapy and energy psychology. After learning that the body holds information about a person from conception onward, and that if this material remains unconscious, destructive behavior patterns, unhappiness, or illness may result, I decided to study this material in more depth, especially the role of anger.

Once I applied and was accepted into the Philadelphia College of Osteopathic Medicine's doctoral program in clinical psychology and behavioral health, I designed a doctoral dissertation that identified and created tools to ameliorate the effects of anger on the body (Wilner 2004). This book, in part, stems from that research. It helped me discover methods to transform anger, preserve health, and contribute to happiness, which are all central themes in this book.

Owning My Own Repressed Anger

This book has a specific focus on helping women, like me, free themselves from anger's negative consequences. I have to admit that the nice, kind person I perceived myself to be masked an angry, spiteful side. Realizing that I could no longer blame my parents for my anger, I took responsibility for it. After all, it was my limbic system, the part of the brain that houses the fight or flight response, that would catch on fire and look for a fight, argument, or chance to get back.

I forever regret the anger I once spat out at a colleague. The situation resolved, after several complaints had been lodged against him, but not without my feeling guilt and shame for blaming him in public. When I was asked to fire someone for unethical behavior, my anger expressed itself driving home, my foot pressing down hard on the gas pedal. The ticket I received for speeding forced me to look at the power of unconscious anger—anger that exists totally out of our conscious awareness. At other times, I suppress my anger. My first marriage ended in divorce because I had not developed the ability to discuss issues that annoyed me. Instead, I turned my resentment inward, allowing it to fester, and wallowed in negative thinking and blame.

Given my life experiences, and my work as a clinical psychologist over the last forty years, my goal in writing this book is to integrate somatic practices with cognitive behavioral therapy (CBT) techniques related to thoughts, feelings, and behaviors. (Beck 1999; Beck 1979; Beck and Freeman 1990). I believe that women, by transforming their anger into a positive force, can communicate rationally and reasonably with those whose views differ from their own and find more love and purpose in their lives.

How You Will Benefit

By following *Releasing Toxic Anger for Women*'s seven-step program, you will:

- Learn body therapy methods that decrease anger and increase pleasure, fulfillment, and happiness

- Create a better energy flow, decreasing stress in your body

- Share angry feelings in a reasonable and rational way, without blame or judgment

- Change negative thinking patterns to positive thought patterns that decrease anger

- Become less reactive to anger directed at you

I encourage you to keep an anger journal as you go through the seven steps. It allows you to map your progress; you can observe your anger change over time. It also gives you a place to write answers to exercises included here so you can keep them all together. There is one additional benefit. An unknown fact about journaling: it's good for your health. People with medical conditions who wrote for at least fifteen minutes several days per week decreased symptoms of depression, felt more hopeful, and made fewer medical appointments (Pennebaker 2003).

Releasing Toxic Anger for Women will help reformat your anger holistically—mind, body, spirit, and emotion. The somatic exercises woven into each chapter are designed to free up anger from places you hold it so that you can use it purposefully and creatively to accomplish your goals. Anger will change from a negative force linked with chaos, revenge, judgment, and destruction to a positive energy flow that enables self-worth, productive thinking, honest communication, and loving relationships. This open-hearted state leads to a realistic view of others, accepting their differences without judgment.

Now it's time to dive in, learn more about your unique brand of anger, and commit yourself to a change process full of fun, challenges, and rewards.

Part 1

THE BASIC PRINCIPLES

CHAPTER 1

Understanding Toxic Anger in Women

When we take responsibility for our hate, our cruelty,
we have...begun the journey of self-transformation.

—John C. Pierrakos, *Love, Eros and Sexuality*

As Danielle explained to me, "I have a problem with anger. I slapped my fiancé over the holidays and almost lost him; I don't want that to happen again. In school, I had temper tantrums and threw books at the teacher. In high school, basketball gave me an outlet for my anger." Danielle is overly aggressive and needs help controlling strong emotions.

Alternatively, anger surges in Linda's chest and her stomach makes a fist, but she perseveres. After biting down on her inner lip to gain control, she says to the client who threatened to take her business elsewhere, "It's fine, I understand." She represents women who suppress their irritation and anger so that negative emotions do not take over their psyche or their lives. But she too needs help. Suppressed anger endangers her health and she lacks communication skills to stand up for herself.

The Difference Between Destructive Anger and Healthy Anger

Taming the anger beast leads to decreased physiological arousal, better health, and authentic communication. But first, we need to understand it better. Women's anger has many faces, including resentment, volatility, destructiveness, aggression, sarcasm, impulsivity, negative thinking, irritation, annoyance, jealousy, envy, criticism, contempt, evil, bullying, and blame. They can vary in intensity from mild irritation or annoyance to intense fury, rage, and hate. Maybe you can relate to one or more of these anger types.

Some anger researchers differentiate anger from hostility, defining *hostility* as an attitude, the desire to hurt someone and get revenge. Feeling vicious or vindictive, you want them to experience the same amount of pain you experienced. *Anger*, accompanied by hormones that cause your body to spring into action, is depicted as yelling, throwing things, withholding, or not talking to someone for one or more days (Spielberger et al. 1983). In this book, I treat hostility and anger as one since they are both controlled by negative thinking and the same biochemistry. Two sides of the same coin, they each have the potential to destroy relationships, initiate or worsen health problems, and discourage authentic self-expression, reparative communications, and optimal self-care—creating chaos in women's lives.

The Effects of Toxic Anger

Toxic anger hurts. We use anger to hurt ourselves and others. Anger lowers self-esteem. We feel ashamed and promise ourselves and the recipient of our anger that it won't happen again, but it does. If we strike out at another, slam a door, yell, throw a plate, pinch, or hit, we feel guilt, self-disgust, and self-hate a few minutes to a few hours later. Unless we confront self-hate and resolve it, inner resentment can last forever, even when it drops out of conscious awareness.

Sometimes we turn anger against our bodies: we stop eating, eat poorly, cut ourselves, use drugs, become couch potatoes, or develop addictions to nicotine, cocaine, or alcohol. Cardiovascular disease, often related to anger, is the number one killer of humans on the planet. Anger has been linked to cancer and heart disease in those who suppress it, as they are too nice to make waves and fight for themselves (Benson and Stuart 1992; LeShan 1977; Powell et al. 1993; Simonton and Simonton 1980; Wolman 1988). In addition to physiological costs, anger has emotional costs; it takes a toll on our relationships.

If after expressing your anger aggressively, or suppressing it in your body, you feel guilt, shame, or low self-esteem, you may become trapped in a vicious circle. First, you respond with anger toward a person or situation. Then, your anger turns against yourself in the form of guilt. Feeling badly, you dump more anger into the world around you, or into your body, which triggers more guilt. You are now caught in a vicious circle.

Here's how a vicious cycle can look. One intelligent, beautiful, creative person I knew erupted when other women appeared to flirt with her boyfriend at the gym. Later, in the women's locker room, she would throw things, stomping around the room. When the attack ended, she collapsed in anguish, apologizing to her friends. After observing this, I described one such incident in my journal:

> *Doris threw her hairbrush at the locker room wall because Gail*
> *smiled at Jim in the swimming pool. It took me an hour to talk her*
> *down and remind her that a smile is not a seduction. Once calm,*
> *she appeared overcome with guilt. Today, she sent me an apology*
> *note that listed the stresses she was under and that she would not*
> *act out again. However, I doubt that will be the case.*

Doris made three mistakes with her anger: one, by being overly dramatic; two, by losing control and throwing things; and three, by turning it into guilt, which produces more anger. Unlike Doris, it's important for you to voice your anger in a clear and reasonable way. You can use the part of your brain that produces anger, the limbic system, to enhance your life and protect yourself, but in a positive, respectful manner.

Basically, anger is a healthy emotion—energetic and alive. It serves the human species well, warning of approaching danger so that we can respond appropriately. It motivates us to react to personal attacks and threats to our security. Anger pushes us to make changes in our lives in order to achieve our goals. When I was trying to sell my house, my realtor failed to hold open houses. Anger motivated me to change realtors and find someone more suitable. Many letters to the editors of newspapers, both local and national, result when we feel wronged. Through anger, we find our voices and publish our grievances. Anger helps us talk to each other; it can create more intimacy. We can use anger to open up a discussion that leads to concessions by both parties. Reflective anger means we take time to think about the problem and do some problem solving. We ask ourselves, *What is the best way to handle this situation?* We can use anger to achieve a win-win for both parties.

To learn more about your anger, do the next exercise. It will help you pinpoint the myriad of situations, people, and events that trigger your anger. Some of these situations produce more anger than others. The anger family includes many feelings, such as resentment, annoyance, irritation, judgment, blame, contempt, hostility, criticism, disgust, rage, violence, bullying, jealousy, hate, and envy.

EXERCISE: My Anger Triggers

Use the following two lists to identify your anger triggers and write them in your journal. If you are reminded of specific people in your life whose behavior fits into one or more of these categories, add their names next to the attribute or behavior. If your triggers aren't listed, add them to the lists. Finally, rank order your top five anger triggers from "makes me most angry" to "makes me least angry."

People who are (traits)...

1. Bullies; put down and demean others

2. Thieves; steal, con, rob, or scam

3. Cheaters; have affairs

4. Rapists, molesters, sexual abusers

5. Accusers; blame, criticize, attack

6. Rejectors; act rejecting

7. Addicts; drugs, sex, alcohol, food, work, nicotine

8. Zealots; religious or political

9. Negative; use bad words, curse, criticize, judge others

10. Hard to hear, whisper

11. Selfish; think only of themselves

12. Unfair, unjust

13. Rude

14. Arrogant; think they're better than others

15. Noisy; shout, loud anger

16. Cruel

17. Pushy and controlling

18. Passive; weak, don't say what they want

19. Dishonest

20. Neglectful

21. Messy, dirty

22. Rigid, compulsive

23. Racist, prejudiced

People who (actions)...

1. Drive slowly, too fast, recklessly

2. Create unnecessary rules and regulations

3. Use bad words, curse

4. Lie

5. Don't listen or pay attention

6. Exaggerate, make up stories

7. Waste time, goof off

8. Keep others waiting, are late

9. Change plans without communicating

10. Falsely accuse

11. Break promises, betray trust

12. Forget birthdays, holidays, and important occasions

13. Work in hospitals or for health care systems that don't deliver

List additional triggers of your anger in your journal. Now rank order your top five triggers from what makes you the most angry to the least angry. Is there a relationship between what triggers your anger currently and events that occurred in your childhood? If so, write about it in your journal.

Understanding Anger's Origins

The thoughts you have when you perceive that you or the people you care about are in danger trigger both anger and fear. However, with fear you experience a lack of control, as if you are at the whim of the situation, whereas with anger you feel in command, empowered, and as if you can personally effect change.

Anger connotes power: it ignites the synapses (nerve endings) in your brain that create the thoughts *I'm in control, I can win here,* or *I will get even*. In less than a thirtieth of a second, these thoughts allow chemicals to release into your blood that prepare you to fight outwardly (get aggressive), fight inwardly (harbor negative, get-even thoughts), or fight sneakily (come up with revenge strategies).

Once they enter your bloodstream, the chemicals make you feel different—unlike your normal self. Perhaps you experience heat, a burning sensation, or your jaw clenches, your eyelids narrow, and your hands tighten into fists. You may direct anger outwardly toward others or inwardly toward yourself—it can go in either direction. And it comes in many variations: vibrant, lively, bitchy, scary, contemptuous, judgmental, aggressive, sarcastic, and even sexy. Or it can be hidden, withheld, vicious, sneaky, passive, and unconscious.

Hidden Anger

Many of you don't want your family members, friends, or colleagues to think of you as angry, negative, or out of control. Therefore, you hide your anger from them and sometimes from yourself as well. You may find yourself saying, "I'm not angry," "I'm fine," or "No worries," even though your gut knots up and unkind thoughts take over your mind. When anger goes unrecognized and unspoken, symptoms develop. For example, you may sweat profusely and have trouble breathing, eating, or sleeping. Or you may have a panic attack because you respond fearfully to the internal experience of anger. Some of you get sick, developing high blood pressure, asthma, rheumatoid arthritis, ulcers, and skin conditions like psoriasis and eczema. Although anger may not be the direct cause of illnesses, research shows that it can make them worse (Banafa, Suominen, and Sipila 2023; Charudhury and Banerjee 2020; Christensen and Smith 1993; Everson et al. 1998; Guidi et al. 2021; Linkins and Comstock 1990).

Toxic Anger

Under normal circumstances, anger is a healthy and even life-saving emotion. It becomes toxic when you respond to uncomfortable or unpleasant events, such as a disagreement between you and your mother, your sixteen-year-old, or your spouse, with aggression and cruelty as if you have to fight to survive. Your brain is perceiving a difference of opinion in the same way as it would view a tiger preparing to attack you in the jungle or a mugger threatening to relieve you of your wallet. You respond with your primitive brain, what Freud called the *id* and Jung the *shadow* (Freud 1960; Zweig and Abrams 1991), rather than your frontal lobes and cerebrum, which control logical thinking and language.

Habitual Anger

When aroused, chemicals pour into your bloodstream that trigger negative behavior patterns that become go-to habits in life. Think of others whose angry behavior is predictable. You know that you can expect rebellion, sulking, distancing, getting back at, destroying objects, or violence from them when they're upset. Due to the guilt factor, you may develop the bad habit of turning anger against yourself: cutting, shaming, or berating yourself and feeling like a bad person. Then, again, if you are a "withholder," habitually suppressing anger for a long period of time, some small, seemingly unrelated event may eventually trigger an explosion.

Transformed Anger

The normal unpleasantries and discomforts of life require good problem-solving skills and coping mechanisms, but not the supreme physiological response and effort that would be appropriate in life-or-death situations. To transform your anger to a positive force, improve your coping mechanisms, and enhance your life, you must come face-to-face with anger rather than dismiss it as a necessary evil or minimize it and pretend that it's not a real problem. Ask yourself to befriend anger, welcome it, and get to know it.

The next exercise provides you with the opportunity to describe your anger. Choose the words that convey how you behave when your anger is toxic, hidden, destructive, or habitual.

EXERCISE: Anger Expression

In your journal, write as many of the phrases below that describe how you express anger.

- Tell others off
- Lecture
- Teach others a lesson ("I'll show you")
- Cool as a cucumber
- Hotheaded
- Act untroubled
- Behave childishly
- Assume an "I don't need you" attitude
- Plan revenge
- Withdraw or distance
- Organize things
- Violent
- Throw or break things
- Work hard
- Nag/nudge
- Throw a tantrum
- Lose control
- Seek control
- Attention-getting
- Behave devilishly
- Cruel
- Blame others

- Bully
- Assume an "I'm right, you're wrong" attitude
- Believe you are owed
- Bitchy
- Deny your anger: "I'm not angry"
- Perfectionism
- Scary
- Sulk
- Don't care what others think
- Look down on others
- Change the subject
- Leave the situation or room
- Aggressive
- Appear troubled
- Mean
- Win at any cost
- "Don't tell me what to do"
- Rebel
- Don't care what you think
- Use other feelings to mask anger
- Throw or break things

The next section introduces you to anger's three main ingredients. To change your behavior, you must treat each separately so that you can control and transform your anger.

The Three-Legged Stool: Anger's Three Components

Imagine your anger as a three-legged stool. The first leg represents your thoughts, the second your feelings, and the third your body and its energy. To transform anger into a positive emotional state, each leg of the stool needs to change.

Your **thoughts**, the first leg of the stool, control how you perceive an event, person, or situation. They also govern your feelings. If another woman were to flirt with your partner, a positive thought such as *That's nice; someone, in addition to myself, finds them attractive* would make you happy. But your inner monster might think, *Who does she think she is? She has no right to look at them like that.* This thought creates anger. Thoughts can take you down one of three paths: negative, positive, or neutral. Your goal is to shoot for 75 percent positive or neutral thoughts per day and reduce your negative thinking to 25 percent or less. According to the National Science Foundation, you have between twenty thousand and sixty thousand thoughts per day and 80 percent are negative, meaning you're thinking negatively way more than positively, and as many as 95 percent of your toxic thoughts are repetitive. Additionally, if you have too many thoughts racing in several directions at once, unless you slow your thinking down and become aware of each thought, as if it were a separate grain of sand, your thoughts will remain clumped together.

Toxic thoughts facilitate aggression, the release of adrenaline and epinephrine, muscle tension, and illness, especially when they are suppressed in your body and not communicated outwardly (Beck 1999; Goleman and Gurin 1993; Goldfried and Sobocinski 1975). Here are some examples of how this works:

- If you overestimate your potential to experience a setback of any kind, you can make yourself sick with worry, anger, or resentment. Joan gave herself an ulcer believing that every time her boss asked to talk to her, he was planning to lay her off.

- Some of you catastrophize, imagining the worst thing that can possibly happen. Georgia presented with panic attacks, explaining that when her boyfriend texted, she envisioned him ending their relationship.

- Others, like Marie, overgeneralize, expecting what once happened to reoccur. The fact that her ex-husband cheated at a conference he attended caused her to rage at her current boyfriend when he signed up to attend a professional meeting.

The exercises in this book, including thought stopping, paradoxical verbalizations, and releasing armor around the heart, will help you transform these thoughts. By perceiving adverse situations differently, you will improve your body's energy flow and substitute positive and neutral thoughts for formerly negative ones.

Uncomfortable *feelings* arise when critical, scary, and negative thoughts tell your brain to send chemicals into your bloodstream. These biochemicals create strange and unpleasant sensations in your body called feelings. They represent the second leg of the stool. Feelings also occur in response to physiological arousal if you perceive yourself to be in danger (Evans 2015). The experience of anger—sometimes known as a secondary emotion because it masks a more vulnerable feeling such as hurt—is often felt in your body. You may report butterflies in your stomach, a tightening in your muscles, or feeling hot all over. Sometimes, when angry, you will endure a heavy or depressed sensation, exhaustion, and difficulty breathing.

Your *body*, the third leg of the stool, receives these chemical messages, or sensations, and prepares to do one of three things in response:

1. **Fight:** You may hold up your middle finger and wave it in someone's face, write an accusatory letter to the editor of your local paper, or roll your eyes at the offending person.

2. **Flee:** You could possibly withdraw, leave the scene, hide, or distance yourself from the source of danger: a behavior called *avoidance* that could include locking yourself away in your room for hours while you harbor negative thoughts.

3. **Freeze:** You may stand still, paralyzed, and like a deer caught in headlights, freeze, hoping to fade into the surroundings so that you will not be seen. In this case fear overrides your anger, but once the fear dissipates, it's necessary to deal with the anger locked away in your body.

In all three instances, your muscles contract and your energy changes from flow to stuck. Holistically, your thoughts, feelings, and body combine and create your behavior—the angry you. To change, it's necessary to separate the parts: your thoughts from your feelings and sensations and both from your body and your actions. The following exercise helps you think about and understand each component.

EXERCISE: The Three-Legged Stool

Think of a recent anger episode and describe the episode in your journal. Then write the first thoughts or images that occurred, the feelings or sensations you experienced in your body, and finally, your behavior: what you did or didn't do. For example,

My seventeen-year-old son got into trouble with the local police for bashing neighbors' mailboxes with a hammer.

Thought: *I have done everything to teach you good values, and you have disappointed me. You're just like your no-good father.*

Feeling/Sensation: *I felt burning in my belly, muscle tension in my neck and upper back, rage, and a desire to hurt him.*

Action/Behavior: *I found myself shouting at him, calling his behavior stupid, and slamming the back door of the house when he returned home.*

Thoughts That Trigger Anger

Descartes said, "I think, therefore I am." He's right, but here's the problem: not all thinking is in your best interest. First, if you overthink and don't give your mind a break, you will burn yourself out. Second, if you have the unique ability to have several thoughts at one time, you will confuse yourself, as the new thought interrupts the previous thought before it's a finished thought. Finally, your brain's main purpose is for solving problems and thinking creatively, not for criticizing and attacking. It has the amazing ability to look at situations and see possibilities and promises. When thinking is filled with blame, judgment, and worry, it leads to toxic anger.

This section introduces you to the kinds of thoughts that are most likely to trigger negativity and anger. They have to do with unmet expectations, unfair treatment, and loss. Thoughts growing out of situations when you are shamed, rejected, or treated as unworthy of love cause pain and resentment. Finally, brutal experiences involving abuse, rape, fear, terror, and victimization facilitate vengeful thinking.

Expectations Unmet

In advice columns such as Dear Abby, parents write that they have stopped talking to adult children who missed Sunday family dinners or failed to make a weekly check-in phone call because their expectations were not met. Customer service representatives leave their jobs when they can no longer tolerate angry criticism from disappointed customers who expected one thing and got another. Women harbor resentment toward those who fail to live up to their promises, such as contractors, manufacturers of products they use, and relationship partners—using anger to avoid experiencing their underlying hurt and disappointment that their expectations were not met. For example,

Julia knew Matt was the one for her. They enjoyed the same bands, laughed at the same jokes, and held a similar work ethic. Matt, who was separated, promised to begin divorce proceedings, but he never

did. After two years, Julia realized that he could not make the break and that her expectations were out of alignment with reality. Furious, anger ate away at her gut, causing gastrointestinal issues.

Thoughts About Unfair Treatment

Women have been victims of injustice. Think voting rights, equal pay, equivalent healthcare, protection against sexual abuse, and entry into certain careers and private clubs. Thoughts about being treated unfairly have inspired you to fight for what you believe is fair. In some situations, you've had to suppress your anger and seethe on the inside. Research reports strong links between cardiovascular disease and perceptions of unfair and unjust behavior (Marmot and Brunner 2005). In Georgia's case,

> Her doctors found it difficult to control her high blood pressure with medication due to unresolved anger about injustice. Her father favored her older sister, Regina, taking Regina with him fishing and leaving Georgia at home. Something snapped when he gave Regina his service medals, prized possessions that Georgia had asked to have. After that, she wanted nothing to do with him, choosing not to attend his funeral when he passed away suddenly. Because she didn't express her anger verbally, it found an outlet in her body.

Vengeful Thinking

Thoughts about not being wanted or accepted lead to vengeful thinking. You have been made to feel undesirable, unlikable, or flawed, and your thoughts go to ways to get back at the person who hurt you. In your mind you seek revenge.

> After she found out that her boyfriend was seeing someone else on the sly—although he was still living with her—Cynthia wanted to get back at him. Feeling unwanted, she asked her friends, "What's

wrong with me?" Bouts of rage replaced feelings of grief and her thoughts flipped to how best to make him hurt. During one fit of rage, she took a rake and scratched both sides of his new car.

Helpless Thoughts

Helpless thoughts bring forth anger and highlight feelings of abandonment, loss, and grief. Once you conclude that you are helpless to change the circumstances surrounding a loss—*No way am I able to affect this situation*—negative feelings take over. Since you can't direct anger toward the object of your loss—perhaps it isn't a person or the person has passed away or left the scene—it spills out onto others or you turn it against yourself. In the next example, the current event brought up unresolved anger and loss from an earlier period.

Nancy's jaw clamped down hard and her fists curled, preparing to punch someone. Through tense lips, she told me that her daughter, a visiting nurse, had been called back to work due to COVID-19. Her negative thoughts focused on household chores that would fall upon her, as she was already overwhelmed by demands from her teaching job. Early images from her past about loss and abandonment were shaping her current reaction. The horror at being left alone in an orphanage when her parents could no longer afford to keep her transferred onto this situation.

Fear and Anger Shout Danger

Some situations produce thoughts that trigger fear and anger, which, like salt and pepper, often occur together, jeopardizing your health (Suinn 2001). If your four-year-old starts to cross a street to retrieve a ball, first you think, *They could be hit by a car*, and feel numbing fear, but a second later you're yelling, "Don't step off that curb, I've told you before it's dangerous, why don't you listen!" Anger tops fear. You may have the same experience in less perilous circumstances, such as when you discover that your secretary forgot to tell you about an important phone call. You think, *I will appear inept to my customers*, and you immediately feel fear, which is quickly covered by anger, and then you make a sarcastic comment to your secretary.

When I asked my colleagues to share their thoughts about the relationship between anger and fear, I received the following responses:

- Being angry is not my primary feeling: It's a behavior for pure protection that overlays fear. When I panic, I notice that fighting and being angry help me survive.

- Sometimes people feel angry because they are fearful and it's hard for them to differentiate their underlying feelings.

- Thoughts about death is the ultimate fear. Anger is energizing and life affirming.

- Fear is an uncomfortable emotion. Your thinking involves admitting a perceived weakness or flaw in yourself.

- Some women have the illusion that fear is weak and anger is strong. Anger feels like power and is driven by thoughts like "I am right," whereas the thinking that corresponds with fear says, "I am vulnerable and weak."

- Fear is harder to allow myself to feel than anger; then I feel helpless and I freeze.

- Deep fears feel life threatening, but anger mobilizes my energy.

Shameful Thinking

Shameful thinking can also trigger anger. It occurs when you regret something you did, thought, or said, because it might make you look "bad" or "stupid." Since you dread appearing ridiculous or weak in other's eyes, you may cover over your shame with anger and blame someone else or yourself for this predicament. Here is an example from my life:

When the supervisor of the clinic where I interned complained to
my dean about my recordkeeping, I felt shame. I did not want to be
caught looking bad. For several months afterward I had vengeful
thoughts and fantasized that she would lose her job.

Thoughts and Trauma

If you have been sexually or physically abused, you have experienced trauma. Trauma causes you to freeze mentally, physically, and
emotionally. During and after those scary moments, your thinking may
be confused, and thoughts may be repressed or forgotten. Meanwhile,
your body is still paralyzed by fear, holding terror and rage toward the
perpetrator within it. Once you feel safe, you can slowly release the
emotions from your body and tell your story. Many of the exercises in
Part 2 will help you release the remnants of trauma from your body.

As you can see, all these thoughts, from unmet expectations to
wanting to get back at someone who shamed you, trigger hurt, fear, and
anger. If you can become aware of them before they cause arousal and
toxic chemistry to release into your body, you will have an opportunity
to transform your anger and move in a positive direction. Try this
thought stopping exercise to get started with this process.

EXERCISE: Thought Stopping

Identify a negative thought that you have often. It can be toward yourself or
someone else, such as "I'm stupid" or "you're stupid." Each time you catch
yourself thinking that thought, visualize a big red stop sign in your mind's
eye or a poisonous insect buzzing around your head. After a few times, that
thought will no longer be a problem. Another option is to drop a quarter in a
jar whenever you have a bleak thought. When the jar is full, donate it to your
favorite charity.

When Anger Backfires

In this chapter, you learned that anger is a normal, healthy emotion that can help you extend your life. You saw how it can backfire and become toxic when fueled by the chemicals that cause physiological arousal. Every angry incident in your life so far has had three facets—your negative thoughts, your feelings, and your body—and combined, they lead to your actions. You also learned that your anger causes you to lose parts of yourself. Other feelings you experience, such as disappointment, fear, shame, grief, and even pleasure, may remain unrecognized because they are overpowered by your anger. As you move on to chapter 2, prepare to focus on the three main anger types and see where you fit best. Stay motivated. Your goal—to change your anger from overly aggressive, or its opposite, unexpressed aggression, to an authentic, positive, and reasonable expression—is in sight. The next exercise will prepare you for the soon-to-come, seven-step anger transformation journey.

EXERCISE: Your Daily Anger Journal

Begin a daily anger journal. Use it at the end of each day to describe your angry thoughts, angry feelings, and angry behavior. Did you lose your temper, attack someone, turn it against yourself, or communicate it rationally? Also use your journal to note changes in how you responded. Perhaps you handled a difficult situation without resorting to criticism or suppressing angry feelings within your body.

CHAPTER 2

Three Anger Types: Discovering Yours

It may be necessary to encounter the defeats, so you can know who you are, what you can rise from, how you can still come out of it.

—Maya Angelou

Your body provides information about you that your brain may or may not know. Whereas your body has experienced every life event since you were conceived and grew in the womb, your conscious memory didn't evolve until age three or later, and it chooses to remember some things and not others. Experts in the fields of behavioral health, somatic therapies, psychology, and psychiatry explain that approximately 50 percent of you is shaped by nurture, what you *learned* from the people who raised you, and 50 percent by nature, what you *inherited* from your genetic line, parents and grandparents (Bouchard et al. 1990). Therefore, your behavior when angry has most likely been influenced by your genetics as well as the treatment you received prebirth, during birth, and after birth. Nurture and nature both have a say about how you act under stress, each contributing to the level of arousal in your body, the amount of adrenaline, noradrenaline, epinephrine, and cortisol (the stress hormones that flow into your bloodstream during an angry episode), and how you react to these chemicals once they invade your bloodstream—particularly if they stick around for a while.

The events and conditions that affected you during infancy and childhood, when your brain was developing—such as the food you ate, the medicines you took, the quality of the air you breathed, and the treatment you received from your caretakers—have also played a major role in how you process, experience, and behave when angry. If one or both of your parents became impatient with you, looked at you with ire, said something nasty, criticized you, spanked you, or abused you, you responded in certain ways. Perhaps your muscles contracted when stress hormones associated with anger and fear poured into your body. Or you may have believed they were right; you really are a bad person. Maybe you felt angry in response, even though you were not aware of it at the time. Other potential responses include willing yourself to feel no pain, crying profusely, apologizing, fantasizing revenge, or making yourself small in order to disappear. It's possible that you also developed allergic reactions or more serious health issues.

Even though the past has passed and is over and done with, your current behavior when angry is partly due to your experience as the recipient of someone else's anger—the brand of anger you received in childhood when your brain and behavior patterns were forming. Sometimes you act exactly like your parents did, copying the behavior they exhibited because that's what you know, and at other times, you make every effort to do the exact opposite.

Because your body has its own intelligence, it can mimic the postures, muscular movements, and behaviors of people who have been in your close orbit. For instance, if you emulated your grandmother and she suppressed her anger or turned the other cheek, you may have trained yourself to follow her lead, and in doing so, you feel closer to her. Or you may have unconsciously copied the behavior of an uncle whose anger frightened you, taking on the behavior that you despised. Although acting like those you dislike, even hate, doesn't make sense, it is a well-known coping mechanism called introjection. You take on negative and toxic behaviors in order to have control over them.

Rather than being controlled by your genetics or past experiences, you can find new ways to deal with anger through this book; but first you need to identify your anger type.

Recognizing Your Anger Type

Learning about your anger type will help you choose the best exercises and techniques to decrease and transform your anger. You will be able to respond rationally to stressful situations in a matter of hours rather than days, weeks, months, or years. By observing your angry self, you will see yourself as others see you when you are unable to control your emotions or when you are keeping them under wraps. The exercises will help you become aware of how anger affects your relationships, find out more about your anger's origins, and seek new ways of dealing with anger rather than repeating the same old unproductive, toxic patterns.

Creating New Patterns in Your Brain and Body

The energy techniques you will acquire in this chapter are used by body and somatic therapists to convert anger from negativity to positivity, and even to love. The underlying theory asserts that life flow is necessary to maintain health and process strong emotions (Pierrakos 1974, 1987). This is similar to acupuncture or any of the Eastern practices based on energy. These techniques assist blocked energy to release back into your body, helping you to establish a sense of inner peace, containment, and body awareness. These exercises have been found to lower blood pressure and increase health when paired with techniques that highlight positive or neutral thought processes (Wilner 2004). You will soon read about how to respond to frustrating situations according to your anger type. Because the three anger types (and their three subtypes) respond to frustrating situations differently (Lowen 1958), the exercises vary depending on the specific behavior to be transformed.

The process, known as *paradoxical movement and thought*, focuses on your habitual, negative, and unconscious patterns before helping you to acquire new, positive ones. It directs you to move your body as you focus on your toxic angry thoughts. These exercises differ from regular exercise routines in that they change your brain as well as your body by helping old attitudes, thoughts, and memories fade into extinction.

The first few times I did these exercises I felt foolish and you may also. If someone were to have seen me stamping my feet and hitting down with my fists, I would have felt embarrassed. However, the results made a huge difference in my life. Find a private space, even if it is a bathroom or a closet, and try the exercises for the types with which you identify.

Helpful hint: If you have children, invite them to do the exercises with you. Children have fun with these exercises, and you will give them the gift of teaching them how to deal with their anger sooner rather than later.

If you feel resistance because the exercises bring back painful memories that you're not ready to face, you may experience a strong desire to stop them prematurely. You may refuse to say the words that go with the exercise or experience an impulse to leave the room to do something else. You may start to laugh. If any of these occur, you are probably close to a truth about your anger that you don't want to admit to yourself. So, if you find yourself saying "no" to the exercise, look within yourself for the courage to overcome your resistance and do the exercise anyway. The results will be worthwhile.

The exercises take only a few minutes per day. They are designed to help you become more aware of your anger, conscious of its origin, and knowledgeable about how it controls your life. They will help you view your anger objectively and transform it from withheld or aggressive to accepting and loving. To do that, it helps to get to know your anger style.

This book focuses on the three main forms of toxic anger and their three subtypes, which are described in the table below.

1. *Anger-Out, Aggressive/Expressive* means that you express anger loudly or aggressively and use it to target other people

2. *Anger-In, Suppressed/Withheld* results when you repress or deny your anger

3. *Passive-Aggressive* anger refers to inconveniencing or making life difficult for the recipients of your anger, although they cannot say with certainty that they have been under attack, and you may not be conscious that you acted out of anger

The Three Anger Types Table

Type One, Anger-Out, Aggressive/Expressive

- *Personality:* Power dynamic, "I am right, listen to me!"

- *Energy:* When angry, energy flows upward in the body—head, neck and shoulders, upper body feels strong, in charge, leadership; Lower body de-energized, less sensation

- *Subtype:* Firecracker

  - *Personality:* Cool, Analytic

  - *Energy:* When angry, highly energized, intense; Quickly dissipates

Type Two, Anger-In, Suppressed/Withheld

- *Personality:* Generous, Wants to be liked

- *Energy:* When angry, energy can be blocked in the mid-section, Body feels sluggish

- *Subtype:* Semi-Rational

  - *Personality:* Achievement oriented, Detaches from negative emotions

  - *Energy:* When angry, has a lot of energy, contains it and maintains it well

Type Three, Passive-Aggressive

- *Personality:* Insecure, Vengeful

- *Energy:* When angry, energy flow blocked, muscles contract, Stays angry longer.

- *Subtype:* Needy

  - *Personality:* Intelligent, Wants justice

  - *Energy:* Varies, highs and lows

Healthy anger, in comparison, implies that you take responsibility for your anger and share your feelings in a reasonable and rational manner with the intent to solve problems and repair your relationship. When you make healthy anger a goal, you can look forward to enhanced happiness, wellness, meaningful conversations, and empowerment.

The three anger types (and subtypes) are described in the next section. Stories illustrating the behavior, told by women whose names and information have been changed to protect their identities, follow each type. As you read about them and try to find yours, know that it's not unusual to identify with more than one type. Some of you may see yourself in all of them, although one is more likely to prevail in certain situations or with specific people. After you have identified your type, complete the associated exercises. If you can't discern where you fit, do the exercises for all of them because they will help you determine your primary anger type. Energy exercises involve the voice and the throat. Vocalizing the assigned words will help you initiate new mental patterns.

Type One, Anger-Out, Aggressive/Expressive

Women's Anger-Out, Aggressive/Expressive behavior involves directing negative vibes, words, and physical aggression toward others by nagging, yelling, attacking, blaming, whining, complaining, throwing things, hitting, spanking, abusing, and using sarcasm and language to reject, judge, criticize or demean. Believing in your rightness, you expect others to agree with you and when they don't, you get angry. Usually your power, natural charisma, and leadership skills help you get your way, but if you encounter resistance or are rebuked or rebuffed, you become aroused. When that occurs, your energy moves up into your shoulders, chest, neck, or head, and you lose some of your natural grounding. Somatic therapists suggest that blocks in your legs and pelvis force energy into your upper body, supporting a fiery anger and a desire for power, status, and success (Pierrakos 1995). To others, you may appear hotheaded, explosive, or scary. Your actions when angry can stem from being on your own as a child and having had to figure things out for yourself. Not believing that the adults in your environment could protect you, you learned to trust your own judgment and take care of yourself. Therefore, you expect others to agree with you and when they don't, your behavior can turn aggressive. This explains Jordan's behavior in the following story:

> *Jordan, a partner in a well-known law firm, joined one of my groups at her partner's request. On the evening of the sixth meeting, I arrived at my office three minutes late due to a traffic jam. Eight group members waited for me to unlock the door, but Jordan wasn't among them. The others explained that she arrived promptly at 7 p.m. and when I didn't, she left without saying a word. Later, I tried to reach her by phone, but she did not return my call. Eventually I ran into her at a local market and she apologized. My failure to live up to her expectations of how a "good therapist" behaves triggered her anger. High arousal made it impossible for her to consider whether I had a valid reason, wait for an explanation, or say goodbye to other group members.*

Women who exhibit Type One, Anger-Out, Aggressive/Expressive behavior may attempt to get back at the person who hurt them. Different from Anger-In, Suppressed/Withheld and Passive-Aggressive types, they don't hide their anger. It's visible for everyone to see.

If you're a Firecracker, a common subtype of Type One, your anger is aggressive and explosive; whereas Type One knows why she is angry, you're out of touch with the cause of your anger. It moves up into your chest and head so quickly that you don't know what triggered it. You feel calm and relaxed, then suddenly you erupt, going from feeling good to feeling like you want to break things in ten seconds or less. Something unexpected overwhelms your nervous system; your body can't hold it and your mind can't control it. But then it subsides as quickly as it came, and you feel like yourself again. Meanwhile, those who observe your anger may feel confused and even scared. This occurred for Kay, when she lost control.

Kay felt overwhelmed. The clock said 6:30 p.m. Late arriving home from work, she found her children watching television, homework undone, and her husband in the home gymnasium being his normal, unhelpful self. The unplugged crockpot meant dinner had not been prepared. As she stirred the soup, a last-minute creation made from yesterday's leftovers, Jeremy, her nine-year-old, came into the kitchen crying. His teacher told him that if he did not bring his field trip money tomorrow, he would not be able to go. Suddenly, she heard herself screaming and shrieking, "Not one more thing, I can't take it anymore. Get out of here! Now! Leave me alone!" Jeremy ran out of the room looking stricken. A few minutes later, Kay stood in the kitchen, shocked by her own behavior; how could she have lost control like that?

Now that you have been introduced to Aggressive/Expressive anger and its Firecracker subtype, do the two exercises that follow.

EXERCISE 1: Paradoxical Movement and Thought

Do the following exercise for two minutes, five days a week for two weeks, and after that, every other day for two additional weeks. Try to do it at approximately the same time every day. Generally, people like to do this exercise first thing in the morning; however, if you have problems sleeping, you may try it prior to going to bed.

1. Stand with your feet shoulder width apart, knees slightly bent and both feet facing directly forward.

2. Begin to stamp your feet, bending your knee, so that you raise each six inches to a foot off the ground.

3. As you stamp, make fists and hit down toward the floor, saying the following three statements out loud, ten times each. You can speak softly or shout, but it is important that you say the words at the same time as you stamp your feet and hit down with your fists.

Words for Anger-Out, Aggressive/Expressive: (1) Do it my way.
(2) I'm right, you're wrong. (3) I don't trust you.

This paradoxical exercise will help you see others as equals and develop trust.

Words for the Firecracker subtype: (1) I am here. (2) I exist.
(3) Acknowledge me.

This paradoxical exercise helps women ground, feel safe, and claim their right to receive equitable treatment.

EXERCISE 2: Containment and Control

This exercise helps you experience your anger but hold back or control your impulse to act. By exposing yourself to anger-producing situations, you will be able to tolerate them in the future without becoming defensive or overreacting.

You play the role of the triggering person and the role of yourself. Think of an unflattering comment you have heard in the past from your ex, parents, or kids—such as stupid, unkind, fat, worthless, mean, ugly, or bad mother. Say this comment out loud, using the tone of voice, gestures, and body posture likely to incite your anger, as you:

1. Stand still and relaxed with feet hip width apart, knees bent slightly, so that you are grounded.

2. Make a fist, hold it up, but don't shake it or hit with it.

3. Take slow, deep breaths and call yourself a name, using a noxious tone of voice, and respond by *not responding*.

4. Do this five times, using a triggering word each time. Do it until you hear the words without feeling aroused or reacting.

Alternatively, ask a friend, relative, adult child, or significant other to call you names or criticize you and respond by not responding or by thanking them for their feedback.

Type Two, Anger-In, Suppressed/Withheld

When you exhibit Anger-In, Suppressed/Withheld behavior, you block its outward expression, repressing it and hiding it from others and sometimes from yourself. Type Two anger includes hostile or negative feelings and thoughts about others or yourself. You visualize acts of revenge, curtailing communication, withdrawing from relationships, and secretly wishing pain on those who hurt you. You hide your anger so well that in some cases you do not appear angry, and, in fact, it may be outside of your conscious awareness.

One difference between Type One and Type Two anger is the time delay. If you are Type Two, you may habitually contain rage, anger, or resentment within your body for days, months, or even years, until you finally explode or get sick. Type Two withheld anger contributes to women's illnesses such as breast cancer and heart disease (Linkins and Comstock 1990; MacDougall et al. 1985; Powell et al. 1993; Simonton and Simonton 1980). If you identify with this type, you don't want to alienate others, or you fear retribution, so you push your anger down beneath the surface. When your body can't store one more angry feeling, you may make a critical or sarcastic comment that causes the other to respond defensively. Now you have the permission to erupt. You obtain the release you need, and in your mind, the other person started the argument.

Because you hold on to your negative emotions, your body may feel heavy, sluggish, tight, or constricted. If overly strict or controlling parents raised you, you didn't want to risk losing their love or support so you withheld or suppressed your anger, but at the same time you resented the lack of freedom. Women who have a strong desire to please others, particularly if they fear rejection or loss of love, often identify with this anger type: holding it in, like Evelyn in the next example, until they explode.

At breakfast, Joe spilled water on the floor in the process of filling the coffee pot. Evelyn, still inwardly seething from yesterday's discussion about finances, commented, "Did you have to fill the pitcher that high?" Hurt by her criticism, he yelled, "Leave if you don't like the way I do things." His overreaction gave Evelyn the opportunity to release her bottled-up anger; she screamed at him, "Stupid monster!" Growing up, Evelyn remembered that her parents forbade temper tantrums and any expression of displeasure. Even though she did not consider herself an angry person, the release felt good.

If you belong to the Type Two, Semi-Rational subtype, you choose to withhold your anger, but you are fully aware of its existence. You contain your anger so that it does not embarrass you or hold you back from achieving your professional goals. You most likely have good organizational skills, enjoy physical activity, and want to succeed. Because image is important to you, you choose to act rationally even when triggered by someone else's bad behavior. When angry, your body tenses, and your voice changes so that it sounds terse or soft. Until you calm down and come up with a solution, you are likely to self-isolate, take a walk, go to the gym, or delve into a work project. Because you, like Lillian in the example below, looked for acceptance and admiration growing up, you abstain from expressing any emotion that could make you look bad in other people's eyes.

Lillian, an avid sailor, went to sea when her anger was triggered. She had given her boss valid feedback after he asked her how he should deal with a difficult client. Rather than receiving the expected thank you, he went ballistic, criticizing Lillian for her lack of support. Hurt and angry, Lillian didn't respond. Instead, she clammed up and withdrew. Being on the water with good friends helped her calm down, even though she was not yet able to talk about the situation or ask for help.

Now that you have been introduced to the Anger-In, Suppressed/Withheld type and its Semi-Rational subtype, do the exercises that follow.

EXERCISE 1: Paradoxical Movement and Thought

Do this exercise for two minutes, five days a week for two weeks, and after that, every other day for two additional weeks. Try to do it at approximately the same time every day. Generally, people like to do this exercise first thing in the morning, however, if you have problems sleeping, you may try it prior to going to bed.

1. Stand with your feet shoulder width apart, knees slightly bent, and both feet facing directly forward.

2. Begin to stamp your feet so that you raise each six inches to a foot off the ground, bending your knee.

3. As you stamp, make fists and hit down toward the floor, saying the three statements out loud, ten times each. You can speak softly or shout, but it's important that you say the words at the same time as you stamp your feet and hit down with your fists.

Words for the Anger-In, Suppressed/Withheld subtype: (1) I won't do what you want. (2) No. (3) Don't tell me what to do.

This paradoxical exercise helps women who withhold negative emotions feel empowered. Women make good choices if they are free to say "no."

Words for the Semi-Rational subtype: (1) I won't show you my anger. (2) You will never know how I feel. (3) I am in control.

This paradoxical exercise helps achievement-oriented women surrender to their feelings and express them.

EXERCISE 2: Authentic Expression

Expressing your anger in a nonconfrontational way is the goal of this exercise. Practice owning your anger, accepting it, and verbalizing it. When you become aware of your anger building, you need to send a signal to yourself to express it verbally. You might pinch yourself or wrap a rubber band around your wrist and snap it. Authentic anger expression involves making "I" statements such as "I feel angry when what I have to say is ignored."

1. First, make an unflattering comment about yourself, one you have heard in the past from your ex, parents, or kids—such as stupid, unkind, fat, worthless, mean, ugly, or bad mother. Use the tone of voice, gestures, and body posture most likely to incite your anger.

2. After calling yourself a name in a noxious tone of voice, stop, experience your feelings, and take slow, deep breaths to calm yourself.

3. Then respond verbally so as not to escalate the situation. For instance, you might say, "When I experience disrespect, I feel angry."

4. Alternatively, ask a friend, relative, adult child, or significant other to criticize you and then respond verbally, trying not to escalate the situation. Example: "That hit below the belt, and it hurts."

Type Three, Passive-Aggressive

Unlike the other two forms of anger, Passive-Aggressive anger is expressed secretly, sometimes unconsciously, and occasionally sneakily. If you want to get back at someone, but you don't want anyone to know you're the culprit, Passive-Aggressive anger is the perfect tool. You may try to make it look like an accident, such as "Can you believe I left my checkbook at my mother's house?" or like you forgot, explaining, "My mind went blank and when I remembered the meatloaf, it was burned to a crisp."

When you want to retaliate, but don't want to take responsibility for your anger, or even admit you have anger, this may be your go-to behavior. You most probably find anger an uncomfortable emotion, but you have a strong need for revenge. Your behavior may be connected to deeper feelings of insecurity and lack of confidence. You may not believe that people will respect you or that you have the right to communicate your anger directly. Sometimes you are totally unaware that you acted out of anger, truly believing that you did indeed forget or that whatever occurred was indeed accidental. In the following story, Suzanna exemplifies this type:

Suzanna's spite and anger hid behind a lovely smile that suggested a comforting and helpful presence. Anger accumulated toward Phil, her live-in partner, who worked long hours at his law firm, leaving her to fend for herself most evenings. Informed that the law association in their city was honoring him for community service, she failed to show up, even though she knew it would mean a lot to him. Forgetting the ceremony, or so she said, she took her sixteen-year-old niece out for ice cream.

If you belong to the Passive-Aggressive, Needy subtype, you feel as if you have been treated inequitably. At some point, you have thoughts like, *You don't listen to me, You don't care about me, You don't understand me,* or *You probably won't remember my birthday.* Early childhood experiences may have led you to believe that your turn will never come. Perhaps you had to care for the adults in your family rather than the other way around. When women can't get what they want and need after years of patiently serving others, then like June, getting even may become the end result.

Behind June's apparent agreeableness hides an almost diabolical need to get back at the mother who neglected her. An only child, her childhood was taken up by her mother's inability to function without June's help. When her mother passed away, she directed her aggression toward women who reminded her of her mother. A female partner in the law firm where she worked particularly irked her. When this woman asked for June's help, things would go awry. Mailing a letter meant losing it on the way to the post office, typing a brief meant delivering the document late, and helping with the company's annual Christmas party meant purchasing the wrong dessert.

Now that you have been introduced to Passive-Aggressive anger and its Needy subtype, do the two exercises that follow.

EXERCISE 1: Paradoxical Movement and Thought

Do the following exercise for two minutes, five days a week for two weeks, and after that, every other day for two additional weeks. Try to do it at approximately the same time every day. Generally, people like to do this exercise first thing in the morning; however, if you have problems sleeping, you may try it prior to going to bed.

1. Stand with your feet shoulder width apart, knees slightly bent, and both feet facing directly forward.

2. Begin to stamp your feet so that you raise each one six inches to a foot off the ground, bending your knee.

3. As you stamp, make fists and hit down toward the floor, saying the three statements below out loud, ten times each. You can speak softly or shout, but it is important that you say the words at the same time as you stamp your feet and hit down with your fists.

Words for both the Passive-Aggressive type and the Needy subtype:
(1) I will get even. (2) It's your fault. (3) It's not fair.

This paradoxical exercise helps women stop blaming and needing to get back at others.

EXERCISE 2: Authentic Expression

This exercise is designed to assist you in sharing angry feelings in a nonconfrontational way. When you become aware of anger building, send a signal to yourself to express it verbally. Pinch yourself or wrap a rubber band around your wrist and snap it. Authentic anger expression involves making "I" statements such as "I feel angry when my contributions to the conversation are ignored."

FINAL CHAPTER EXERCISE: What Form Does My Anger Take?

The following self-assessment helps you determine your anger type. Is your type (1) Anger-Out, Aggressive/Expressed, (2) Anger-In, Withheld/Suppressed, or (3) Passive-Aggressive (getting back without being found out)?

In your journal, record as many forms of anger listed below that you experience currently or have experienced in the past. Write the letters that best describe your anger type next to the form your anger takes—A/E for aggressive, expressed Anger-Out; W/S for withheld, suppressed, unconscious, Anger-In; and P/A for Passive-Aggressive anger.

_____ anger	_____ rage	_____ demean
_____ annoyance	_____ violence	_____ disgust
_____ nervous	_____ critical	_____ displeasure
_____ empowered	_____ guilty	_____ inappropriate
_____ hate	_____ greed	_____ evil
_____ belligerent	_____ jealousy	_____ destructive
_____ bitter	_____ burdened	_____ cruel
_____ intense	_____ quarrelsome	_____ inhospitable
_____ resentment	_____ reject	_____ impolite
_____ stress	_____ judgmental	_____ rude
_____ envy	_____ inflexible	_____ sarcastic
_____ irritation	_____ ferocious	_____ mean
_____ cynicism	_____ vicious	_____ bullying
_____ hostility	_____ blame	_____ self-sabotaging
_____ vengeful	_____ self-righteous	_____ contempt
_____ authoritarian	_____ reckless	

Learning from Your Anger Type

If you were able to identify with one or more of the anger types described in this chapter, you will be more conscious of your anger and able to view it in a new way. Now it will be easier to transform; you will choose exercises designed for you. This chapter has set you on the road to freedom from unhealthy, toxic anger patterns. You've experienced stuck energy begin to move in your body and become aware of your negative thinking. The next section, part 2, will introduce you to the seven steps that will help you release and transform your anger so that you can free yourself from negative thinking, let go of unnecessary stress, and live life fully.

Part 2

SEVEN STEPS
to TRANSFORM
ANGER

Aware: Sensing Your Body's Energy

Man is a multi-sensorial being. Occasionally he verbalizes...

—Ray L. Birdwhistell

Jennifer was asked to withdraw from a sketching class because she was overheard making disparaging remarks about the teacher. She believed the administration treated her unfairly, but she told her closest friend, "I'm not angry. I'll just enroll at another art school." Meanwhile, she could no longer sleep through the night.

Anger doesn't knock on the door and announce itself. How does Jennifer know that she's not angry? Perhaps she simply isn't paying attention to symptoms signaling that an emotional reaction has occurred. It takes awareness to tune in to your body's messages. Do you know when you're angry?

You may be aware of situations in which your teeth clench, your jaw tightens, your face flushes, and your stomach contracts without knowing that each of these physical reactions is associated with anger. You may rush around eighteen hours a day, from activity to activity, repressing irritation, resentment, and rage, shoving them down deep into your body. If you learned as a child that anger is wrong and dangerous, you likely hide your anger in your body where it can't be seen or heard. By blocking these emotions, you send them to live outside your conscious awareness. But they are still there and will pile up. Here is how Camille experienced suppressed anger:

Raised by an ultrareligious and abusive mother who couldn't tolerate anyone questioning her judgment, Camille learned to keep her thoughts to herself. After being slapped across the face for offering an opinion, she bit down on her lips whenever she disagreed with her mother's point of view. Now she does the same thing with her husband. Because she's unable to share her opinions if they differ from his, resentment builds up inside her and she wants to scream. Our work with her suppressed anger began with developing body awareness. When asked to describe the sensations in her feet, she looked down at them and said, "I don't know." Then she said, "Tight," most likely describing her shoes. When asked more questions about her sensations, Camille looked upward as if to solicit answers from the sky. She was unable to connect with her body and the information it could provide her.

Without body awareness, you may live in your head, out of touch with your emotions and feelings. Overfocusing on your thoughts and overvaluing them leads to mistakes in judgment. Thoughts sometimes highlight personal biases and wishes, overlook facts, or they cause you to mistakenly believe you can think your way through all of life's challenges. You can get stuck in a cycle of endless thinking, rumination, and dwelling on fears and anxieties. Overanalyzing past events and conversations may cause you to lose touch with your authentic, in-the-moment experience. If you favor logic, because you think emotions are bad or scary or make you appear weak, you will find yourself out of touch with your body, where your feelings reside. Then, emotions like anger will control you rather than the other way around.

But if you realize your body is a rich and fertile ground for feelings, and like an emotional garden, it grows flowers of every shape and size, you will soon have a different relationship with your anger. For it can be both a beautiful flower that protects you from danger and a poisonous weed when used destructively. This step, *Awareness*, helps you identify the physical sensations that occur with anger and its variations: resentment, disgust, annoyance, irritation, hostility, guilt, jealousy, and rage.

By developing greater awareness, you will learn where you hold anger in your body. Most importantly, you will get in touch with aspects of anger that are hard to access through talk or exercise alone so that you can work with them and transform them. Women have many reasons to be angry, from injustice to lack of control, so by understanding your anger, perceiving it in your body, and grasping how it affects your health and your relationships, you can use it to empower yourself, build bridges, and facilitate positive connections.

The Price of Detaching from Your Body

When you are angry, adrenaline and norepinephrine enter your bloodstream, causing sensations that may make you uncomfortable, that you can't control. If you detach from your body, rather than becoming aware of what is occurring internally, you set yourself up for toxic anger. The actions that result will be guided by physiological arousal rather than rational thought. Then you might attack, or you may hide. Neither resolves your feelings or the problem at hand.

If you're totally oblivious to what goes on in your body and unaware that you feel angry, you pay a price:

- You have no way of handling strong emotions; they control you and you are at their whim. You can't stop or change whatever is happening in the moment.

- You lack warning signs to tell you that you might fly off the handle at any moment, hide under the covers and disappear, or allow someone to override your opinion or boundaries. It becomes too late to change your behavior.

- You put your health at risk because not sensing the adrenaline that stays in your body for too long, or a rise in your blood pressure or heart rate, means that you cannot apply remedies that preserve your well-being.

- You are unable to communicate your anger rationally, come up with a compromise, or work through the problem.

- You are not fully present and therefore less likely to communicate your authentic experience.

To heal toxic anger and make anger work for you—through appropriate communications and positive thinking—you must cultivate awareness. You may experience it as a *felt sense*, a language the body speaks in words or images, to describe authentic emotions being held in your muscles and organs (Gendlin 1978). With the following exercise, I invite you to experience your body's language of sensations.

EXERCISE: Tuning In to Sensations

To identify and sense anger, you must first attune to sensations of every kind. This body scan exercise helps you develop an awareness of physical sensations such as tingling, warmth, pulsating, tightness, coldness, pain, tension, and heat. You may find that some parts of your body feel numb or lack sensation as well. See the illustration Developing Body Awareness.

1. Sit in a comfortable chair or lie down on a mat or bed. Focus on your breathing. Breathe in...and out...naturally. Allow each breath to come and go without any effort to change it.

2. Notice your lungs. Do they fill with air when you breathe in and release fully when you breathe out? Is your breathing shallow or do you take full, deep breaths?

3. Let the lids of your eyes shut and experience the feeling of your eyelids as they close.

4. Sense your shoulders. Do they feel tight or relaxed? Are they pulled up around your ears or dropped down and at ease?

5. Move down to your right foot and scan it for sensations and feelings. Become aware of your right calf, then scan slowly up to your right

knee and right thigh. Feel every sensation. If you don't feel anything, that's okay. Give yourself permission to not feel.

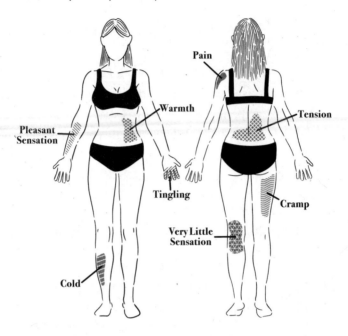

Pain

Warmth

Tension

Pleasant Sensation

Tingling

Cramp

Very Little Sensation

Cold

Developing Body Awareness

6. Next, scan all of the sensations in your left foot, your left calf, left knee, and your left thigh. Bring awareness and a desire to know what is occurring in your left leg and foot.

7. Now, turn to your hips and pelvis. Are there sensations in your hips or under your backside?

8. Move further up; feel into your belly, your stomach, and your gastro-intestinal tract. Notice sensations in your belly, a place where many people hold strong emotion.

9. Come up to your chest and experience your heart and your lungs. Feel into each, asking what you sense there. Envision your heart, whether it's small or large, tight or relaxed, pulsating or expanding. Sense your lungs and feel your diaphragm moving up and down.

10. Experience your back and your spine. Does your lower back feel different from your upper back? Do you have backaches or pain? Does your spine feel strong or weak?

11. Move into your right hand, wrist, elbow, arm, and shoulder. Bring awareness and a gentle curiosity to the sensations in your entire right arm and hand.

12. Scan for sensations in your left hand, wrist, elbow, arm, and shoulder. Continue to bring awareness and a gentle interest to the left arm and hand.

13. Move to your face. Feel the sensations in your jaw, your mouth, around your eyes, your nose, and your ears. Does your face radiate sadness, bitterness, happiness?

14. Notice the back of your head and bring awareness to the top of your head.

15. Notice your throat and neck. Do they seem connected to your body, to your head? What does it feel like to swallow? Is your neck tense or stiff?

16. When you are ready, open your eyes and come back into the room. Be gentle with yourself. Look around and connect with objects in the room.

Write in your journal a description of what you observed about your body's sensations during the scan. Or draw a picture mapping your sensations, similar to the illustration Developing Body Awareness.

I suggest you scan your body daily for the first week, and after that, two or three times a week. Developing awareness takes practice, so the more you tune in to your body, the quicker a sensitivity to its inner workings will develop. A body scan is considered a mindfulness exercise because it requires you to stay present to your experience as it unfolds. Mindfulness, along with energy and relaxation, are covered in the next sections. All three will help you improve your body awareness.

Mindfulness and Anger Awareness

When you live in your head, your thoughts keep you looking back toward the past or forward toward the future. This keeps you away from the present where emotions and authentic experience occur, making it more difficult for you to experience your anger and the circumstances feeding your arousal. Mindfulness means that you welcome your full emotional experience and stay present with it (Hahn 1975; Kabat-Zinn 2013). Being mindful calls you to accept your anger, treat it as a friend, breathe into it, observe it, and appreciate how it feels in your body without changing it, suppressing it, or acting on it.

When you are mindful of your anger, you are in touch with your truth. But women have been taught to ignore their anger and forced to live inauthentically—by parents, churches, and their cultures. Because you have learned to block your anger, hide it, squelch it, and act like it does not exist, you don't respond appropriately when an assertive stance is needed. Consider the following example. Mary needs to practice mindfulness in order to know her anger, accept it, and respond from a position of authority and responsibility.

Mary lived and competed in a man's world. As vice president of finance in a Fortune 500 company, men reported to her. Occasionally, she was discounted or disrespected in meetings. Then she would start to tear up and run to the ladies' room to hide her tears. She told me, "I was taught that negative thoughts were wicked. So I could never be angry." Not being able to handle anger and stand up for herself was a problem.

With mindfulness, Mary learned to experience her anger, feel the edges of it, the shape of it, the color of it, the smell of it, and its intensity. Eventually, she learned to accept it, respect it, share it, and even enjoy it.

My first mindfulness exercise involved a raisin, but it taught me the usefulness of applying it to an emotion like anger. To have the full raisin experience, I had to put it in my mouth and hold it there for several minutes, sensing and tasting, then chewing and swallowing at a very slow speed (Kabat-Zinn 2013). This exercise shows how any object of focus offers sensations that invite us into our bodies to experience them in the present moment.

When you use anger as a focus of your mindfulness, I suggest that you stay with your experience of anger until your body sensations soften and disappear—it may take minutes or hours. For example, if your stomach burns when you're angry, explore and experience the burning sensation until it dissipates. Because you don't act on it, the emotion may be fleeting. But even if it stays longer than you might wish, if you stick with the awareness of your discomfort, you will find that you are able to deal with it.

Once you become mindful of your anger, it begins to change. This is something you can only discover by experiencing it. Do the following mindfulness exercise to help you develop a deeper awareness of anger sensations in your body.

EXERCISE: Mindful Anger

1. Sit or lie in a comfortable, relaxing place.

2. Imagine a closet with a shelf at the top. Put your current thoughts on the shelf and label them so you know what they are in case you want them back. Shut the door to the closet.

3. Paying attention to your breathing, each in-breath and out-breath, breathe slowly and deeply, allowing your breath to take you deeper into your body: into your chest, your spine, and your belly. Now feel it in your pelvis, your legs, and your feet, down to the tips of your toes.

4. Think of a minor irritation you have experienced recently. This should not be something that causes you a lot of distress. Instead, explore your anger through a minor event. Remember what occurred, see it, and hear it in your mind's eye.

5. Continuing to breathe slowly, taking deep breaths in and out, focus on this feeling of anger. Ask where you feel it in your body. Stay with the emotion, observe it, and appreciate the experience of the felt

sense of it in your body. Although these feelings may be uncomfortable, staying with the discomfort will allow you to change.

6. Stay with the sensations until something in you seems to shift or let go.

Write in your journal where you experienced the sensations in your body. If you did not feel anything, write about that as well.

Mindfulness helps you recognize anger before you act on it in ways that can jeopardize your relationships and your health. The next section discusses energy, providing you with an alternative way to become conscious of your anger—through energy flow.

Energy Flow and Anger Awareness

There are many terms for the body's energy, including *chi* in China and *prana* in India. The concept of the body's energy has been used for thousands of years in many healing systems. Thoughts and feelings cause energy to change: Negative thoughts such as "I'm no good" or "You're no good" make it heavy and dense, whereas positive ones such as gratitude create light and vibrant energy. Anger, which is on the negative side of the spectrum, causes heavy and dense energy that gets stuck in the muscles of the body (Brennan 1988; Pierrakos 1987).

You may have noticed that when you are around angry people, their anger seems to poison the air you breathe. The atmosphere in the room becomes inhospitable and you can't wait to leave. I can remember asking the hostess to change my seating in a restaurant because the older couple dining near me were looking at each other with such hostility that I knew I would not be able to enjoy my meal. The same thing happens in your body when you are angry. Your energy contracts, becoming tense and uncomfortable. Sadly, you may be more aware of the toxic consequences of anger when you are around other people's anger than your own, which is why perceiving the energy in your body is so important.

By sensing energy, you can become aware of the places in your body where you hold anger. You may, for example, discover a stiff neck, iron-clad shoulders, an aching lower back, or numb thighs. Knowing when your energy flows well and when it's blocked or cumbrous helps you become aware of being angry. This next exercise will help you to experience the difference.

EXERCISE: Heavy Versus Light Energy

First, imagine something that makes you feel sad and angry: for instance, the death of a favorite pet, the loss of a job you really liked, or a lower grade on a test than you felt you deserved. Sit with that image and those sensations for a full minute or more.

Then do the opposite: visualize a wondrous moment, perhaps dancing in your lover's arms, being on a winning team, or your friends coming through with the best gifts on your birthday. Again, sit with these sensations for a full minute or more.

Write about this experience in your journal. Did the energy in your body change when the image shifted? How was it different?

Blocked energy signals anger. You can locate energy blocks in your body in the ways indicated in this next exercise.

EXERCISE: Awareness of Energy Blockage and Flow

When your anger is stuck and blocked in muscles, that part of the body may lack sensation or be painful. Here are five descriptions you will use in this exercise:

1. *No feeling*, or a lack of sensation, which means that the energy is more blocked than flowing and blood flow into this section is blocked.

2. *Pain* or *tension*, which means that the blood and energy are attempting to move into a blocked section, causing discomfort and pain.

3. *Breathing in and out*, places where the breath can't travel, which reflect blockages and potentially hold anger.

4. *Energy flow*, which means that this body section feels alive and flowing, embraces a feeling of warmth, subtle movement, slight tingling or vitality, and doesn't appear to have any blocks.

5. *Do not know*, which means you aren't sure.

Use these five options to describe your energy in each of the following seven sections of your body. Take a moment, close your eyes, and feel into each area. In your journal, write the number, from 1 to 5, that best describes what you experience next to each body section.

- Top of head, forehead, and eyes

- Mouth, jaw, and chin

- Throat, tongue and neck

- Shoulders, arms, hands, upper chest

- Diaphragm, solar plexus, and middle back

- Abdomen, belly, sacrum, and lower back

- Pelvis, genitals, thighs, calves, ankles, and feet

Let's continue building your awareness of the seven areas of your body that Wilhelm Reich, a disciple of Freud and the father of body therapy and energy psychology in the Western world, defined as energy sections (Reich 1972). Whereas Freud called life energy *libido*, Reich called it *orgone*. Both associated energy with sexuality, physical health, vitality, and emotional wellness.

EXERCISE: Journey Through the Sections of the Body

You can develop awareness of the role anger plays in your body by moving through Reich's seven sections. The italicized subtitles and the descriptions that accompany each section come from my studies and research in energy psychology.

Lie on your back on a comfortable bed or mat and give full attention to your body. Take three deep breaths, exhaling completely, and let go of any tension you are holding. Experience your out-breath carrying negative thoughts and feelings far away and your in-breath bringing you peace and relaxation. At the end of the exercise, write in your journal what you observed on your journey through the seven sections of your body.

1. Top of Head and Eyes: *Wisdom, Spirituality, and Perception.* Sense the top of the head and forehead and ask yourself what you feel. Do you have tension from bouts of negative thinking, anger, worry, or judgments of yourself and others? Is the top of your head relaxed and open to a soft and vibrant energy flow?

Now experience your eyes. What words describe them? Do your eyes jump ahead and attempt to see what will happen in the future? Are they frightened, tired, or hostile? Did you see something noxious in childhood that caused your pupils to contract? Do they turn inward, away from the outer world? Are they vague and absent; hard, cold, mean, and angry; or compassionate, kind, and vulnerable?

2. Mouth, Jaw, and Chin: *Need Fulfillment and Pleasure.* Move lower in your face and sense your mouth and jaw. As you focus on your mouth, notice whether it feels contented or disappointed. Feel your lips. Do you experience them as full or thin? Do the corners of your mouth seem to turn up or down?

Become aware of your jaw; is it tight or relaxed? Do your teeth grind against each other? The jaw may hide the forbidden desire to bite someone or anger from the past that you were prohibited from expressing. You may sense aggression and stubbornness, and an unwillingness to take "no" for an answer in your jaw. Do these parts feel fulfilled and bring you pleasure or is there a sense of unfulfilled needs?

3. Throat, Neck, and Tongue: *Receiving Love and Speaking the Truth.* Now move your awareness to your throat, neck, and tongue. Starting with your throat, envision it as a tunnel between your head and chest. Sense whether it is blocked or open. Contractions and tight muscles in the throat keep emotions like anger that you don't want to express stuck in your body. Besides impeding the expression of anger, the throat and tongue, when blocked, stop you from receiving positive feelings. Love, like food, flows in through the mouth. If you believe you don't deserve affection or support, you may create a throat block.

Bring awareness to your neck; notice whether it's stiff, tense, or relaxed. A stiff or tense neck can mean a need for control, which can lead to anger when you can't control your environment.

4. Shoulders, Arms, Hands, Upper Chest, Upper Back: *Connection to Others, Aggression and Anger.* Bring your awareness to your shoulders, arms, hands, upper chest, and upper back. Does this area feel alive, dull, or even numb? Experience your shoulders' shape and size. Do they feel broad, heavy, light, muscular, collapsed, tight, flexible, relaxed, or contracted? Do they round forward to protect your heart? Are they weighed down with too much responsibility or too many burdens? Do they pull back to imply strength, power, and a desire to have the upper hand?

Flexible and relaxed arms and hands want to connect to others whereas stiff arms and hands held close to the body can express social discomfort, a need to distance from others, or a fear of losing control. Tightly held, muscular arms or hands that curl into fists show aggression and anger.

5. Diaphragm, Solar Plexus, Middle Back: *Represents Living and Breathing Fully.* Bring awareness to your solar plexus, diaphragm, and middle back. Does this area feel alive or lack sensation? The middle of your body concerns achieving your life goals. If your middle is confused, vacant, disturbed, or angry, you may be unclear about your goals or feel frustrated or thwarted—something is blocking your way forward. On the other hand, if this area feels full and alive, life is meaningful, and you are on the path to fulfillment. When the diaphragm moves easily up and down you are most likely in touch with your emotions. Awareness of this section tells you if you have the right to live authentically and to be yourself.

6. Abdomen, Belly, Sacrum, Lower Back: *Power, Creativity, and Self-Care.* Sense what is occurring in your belly, sacrum, and lower back. Do you feel overly full and uncomfortable, blocked, numb, or calm and alive? This area of your body reflects power, creativity, and gut instinct. Your abdomen can collect and hold unwanted feelings, particularly anger. Discomfort in the lower back or sacrum can mean you need more self-care. You may be burnt-out, emotionally exhausted, or recovering from an illness. Do you allow yourself to be powerful, creative, or do you diminish yourself and minimize your needs? Can you fully express your gut's anger, but in a rational, reasonable way? Can you be assertive and set boundaries?

7. Pelvis, Genitals, Buttocks, Thighs, Calves, Ankles, and Feet: *Safety and Security, Sexuality, and Life Energy.* Bring your awareness to your pelvis, hips, buttocks, thighs, legs, and feet. Notice how they feel: shapely, muscular, solid, weak, or collapsed? Do you experience vitality, life, and flexibility in these parts of your body? Do they hold anger? A flexible pelvis welcomes pleasure, whereas a contracted, tight, or armored one fights against it. Legs and feet indicate how you move in life, whether you move forward, regress and move backward, or get stuck in the muck. They also signal how safe and secure you feel on the planet.

As you assess the vitality of each of the sections listed above, try to determine whether energy is flowing or blocked. Now write in your journal a short description of any awareness you received, and whether anger—current or past—may be residing in this section of your body.

The exercises in this step help you increase your ability to sense anger in your body. So far you have learned about mindfulness and energy. Relaxation is the third path to anger awareness. Relaxation exercises help you discern the difference between peace and calm and anger and its companion, tension.

Relaxation and Anger Awareness

If you are relaxed, you cannot feel tense or angry since relaxation and physical arousal are mutually exclusive. Anger causes your body to tense up. If you're angry a lot, tension starts to feel normal. By learning to experience relaxation, you'll know what it feels like to be calm and at peace with yourself, and how these feelings differ from tension and anger. The exercise that follows, progressive muscle relaxation, helps you make this distinction so that you will easily identify your physical state (Jacobson 1938; 1976). During the exercise you may find that some body parts are relaxed whereas others seem overly stressed.

EXERCISE: Progressive Muscle Relaxation

Before you begin this exercise, think of a recent stressor in your life: something or someone who aggravated you or "pissed you off." During this exercise, focus on the sensations in your muscles to learn how your body reacts when it is relaxed versus when it is stressed. Tense only the muscle group assigned, keeping your other muscles relaxed or neutral. Practice this exercise for ten minutes once a day for two weeks. Once you build a body memory of how relaxation feels, your goal is to return to this state whenever you feel tense or angry (Craske and Barlow 2006). You may make a tape of these instructions and play it as you do the exercise, but remember to practice without the tape so that you may do the exercise whenever you have a need.

1. Sit comfortably with closed eyes and a quiet mind.

2. Make fists and pull up on the wrists, creating tension in your lower arms. Experience the tightening from the lower arm down to the fingers. Focus on the contraction and the feeling of discomfort. Hold this position for fifteen seconds and release, allowing your hands and arms to relax with palms facing down. Focus on the warm sensations that now inhabit this part of your body.

3. Create tension in your upper arms by straightening and tightening your entire arm against the sides of your body. Feel the tension flow up the back of the arms into your shoulders and back. Hold this position for fifteen seconds, focusing on the tension. Let the arms release from your sides and experience relaxation, heaviness, and warmth.

4. To tense your lower legs, point your toes up toward your face. Experience your feet and calf muscles contract. The tension encircles your feet, spreads around your toes, and then moves up your legs. Focus on the contraction for fifteen seconds and then release, letting your legs collapse and relax. Experience the comfort and warmth.

5. To create tension in your upper legs, bring your knees together so that they touch and raise your legs off the mat or floor. Focus on the tightness in your hips, down to your upper legs for fifteen seconds.

Release the tension and allow your legs to drop down heavily. Experience relaxation replacing the tension and feel the difference.

6. Pull your stomach in toward your spine and make it very tight to build tension. Focus on the contraction for fifteen seconds. Now let the stomach release and feel the sense of warmth circulating across your stomach. Delight in the comfort of relaxation.

7. Take a deep breath in and hold it to expand your chest and build up tension. Feel the tension spreading from your front to your back. Hold your breath for ten seconds. Exhale and breathe normally, observing the difference between a tense and a relaxed chest.

8. Visualize your shoulders being pulled up around your neck on a marionette's strings. The tension flows down from your shoulders, toward your back, and up into the back of your head. Focus on this contraction for fifteen seconds and then relax, lowering the shoulders to their normal position. Focus on comfort and warmth.

9. Pressing your neck back into your chair or mat, point your chin down toward your chest. Feel the tension at the back of your neck for fifteen seconds and release, letting your head fall back and relax.

10. Clench your teeth and force your lips to turn upward so that your mouth, jaw, and throat tighten. Hold this position for fifteen seconds and then release it, letting your mouth drop open and the muscles around the throat and jaw relax. Feel the difference between the two positions.

11. Close your eyes and squeeze them tightly for ten seconds. Release and let the tension dissipate. Sense the difference when the eye muscles relax.

12. Build up tension in your forehead, raising your eyebrows up as high as you can. Experience the tight pulling sensations across your forehead and the top of your head. Hold for fifteen seconds and relax so that the tension releases and sensations of relaxation takes its place.

13. Finally, create tension in your whole body by tightening every muscle from the toes up to the top of your head. Squeeze everything as tight as you can and hold for fifteen seconds. Now release and let the tension dissipate. Stay in this relaxed state for at least two minutes.

In your anger journal describe your experience. What parts of your body were difficult or easy to relax? Were you able to experience the difference between relaxation and tension? In a few words, describe each state.

Awareness Is Where It Begins

Awareness is where anger transformation for women begins. If you don't know you're angry, you are not going to be able to change it. Or if you know you're angry, but are self-righteous about it, thinking, *I have every right to be angry*, you still need more awareness to discover how your anger is hurting yourself as well as others. By following along with the exercises that are based on well-documented approaches from the fields of mindfulness, energy psychology, and relaxation, you become actively aware of the physiological manifestations of your anger. The knowledge you gain by listening to your body will allow you to change your anger so that it works for you rather than against you. The next step, *Uncover*, will help you find its roots in order to transform it.

Uncover: Discover Your Anger's Source

Until you make the subconscious conscious, it will direct your life.

—Carl Jung

Carina's excessive, out-of-control anger resulted in the loss of colleagues, family members, and partners. Her adult sons threatened to stop talking to her unless she got her anger under control. She carried the rage in her body; anger so bad, she wore her teeth down, grinding them against each other. She knew nothing of the anger's origin, initially telling me she had a close to perfect childhood. Once she recalled experiences from her childhood that she had blocked from her memory, uncovering the root of her anger, she could own her anger.

When she accepted her vengeful self, I had a dream that vividly illustrates how anger imagery can appear in the unconscious. Carina was astride a large alligator, riding him hard, her long golden hair flowing behind her. Her arms held the reins and directed its movements. Its mouth was snapping. She rode it like a crazy child, but she had it under control. When it turned its head and snapped at her, she wasn't afraid. Later, she visited its lair, faced it head on, fed it, and cleaned its mouth. This dream shows Carina learning to control her anger, accept it, embrace it, and work with it. As she did, she could begin to come to terms with her feelings about her abusive, alcoholic father that had haunted her from age six.

When I think about the hundreds, if not thousands, of people I have worked with over the years in workshops, seminars, and therapist training programs, most everyone found the roots of their anger hidden in forgotten or suppressed memories. Whether you yell, scream, slam doors, break plates, threaten others, pout, feel victimized, burn up inside, criticize others, resort to passive-aggressive behavior, or go off by yourself, you step away from negativity and step toward reclaiming your authentic self by finding the origin of your anger and bringing it into conscious awareness.

The goal of step two is to help you quickly discover the source of your anger. To break toxic, unhealthy, stress-laden, and repetitive patterns, it is necessary to go back in time and uncover the event or situation at the point of origin. I understand that you may not want to delve into situations and circumstances that were, at best, unpleasant, and at worst, terrifying. You might even prefer that I offer you positive affirmations, such as "I am full of love and forgiveness," to say whenever you feel irritated or annoyed. Many self-help gurus want you to believe that you don't have to deal with your negative past or painful emotions, but I have not found affirmations to work unless they are paired with letting go of toxic anger that you have held on to far too long.

Identifying your toxic anger's origin is a bit like the game hide-and-seek. Remember when you almost gave up because no matter where you looked, you couldn't find your friend's hiding place. The roots of your anger are similarly well hidden, covered over with loads of psychic debris. Therefore, you may need to employ several of the methods described in this chapter to uncover them. Since your anger originated a long time ago to protect you from pain, you will be excavating layers of life experience to find the original source.

Repeating Toxic Patterns

You may have heard the saying "what you don't know won't hurt you." With toxic anger the opposite is true: "what you don't know *will* hurt you." If you don't know why your anger exists, you will most likely continue to repeat the same patterns. However, by finding its source, you will respond differently. You won't copy the cruel and unacceptable behavior of those who caused you pain, and you will refrain from judgement, criticism, and blame. Whether you are a rageaholic or an anger suppressor, your behavior will change when you discover its roots and engage in habit-breaking, mind–body interventions.

Angry behavior is like being on a carousel with posed horses painted in many different colors that keep spinning around and around. Whether anger is suppressed, expressed, or passive-aggressive, you get on and keep riding the same horse, doing and saying, or not saying, the same things, producing the same painful and disastrous results. Once you uncover the source of your anger, you can get off the carousel and move forward, freeing yourself from the bonds of denial and repetitive patterns. The following exercise will help you do that by tuning in to memories stored in your unconscious.

EXERCISE: Peeling the Onion

Memories pile one on top of another, in layers, like an onion. By starting with more recent memories, you may elicit information about the roots of your anger in the past. Write the answers to the following four questions in your anger journal. If you can't remember, make up an answer because some truth lies within your imagination. Writing about the source of your anger helps you gain distance from the pain associated with it and achieve an objective view of what may have occurred.

1. Look around the room. Pick an object that reminds you of a negative event, situation, or person from the past. Welcome any feelings that occur. Describe this memory in your journal in detail.

2. Focus on the first house, apartment, or dwelling that you remember living in. Ask yourself who lived with you, what your home looked like, where you slept, and where you ate. Did you have a particular place at the dinner table? Did the family eat together? Did you share a bedroom? Draw a picture of the floor plan as well as the outside of the

building in your journal. You don't have to be an artist—stick figures will do. As you remember more about your early years, write about memories associated with anger in that setting.

3. Picture your nursery school, kindergarten, elementary school, junior high school, or summer camp. What was your worst school or camp experience, the most shaming, the most stressful, the most violent? What were the names of your favorite or most detested teachers? Were you the teacher's pet, the class clown, the wallflower, or the bully? Write the memories associated with anger in your journal.

4. Finally, describe a situation in which your behavior reminded you of the behavior of a person from your past who you found repugnant. Describe that person's behavior and how it hurt you. What occurred when you found yourself behaving like that person?

Now that you have looked for the source of your anger in the past by unburying memories, you might recognize that you carry some information about its source in your body as well. Even as you read this, you may find your jaw clenching or your shoulders tensing.

Hiding Within Your Body

Research shows that the unconscious is not some hocus pocus, mysterious place. Instead, your body's muscles, organs, posture, and overall shape and size hold all the information about you that your mind does not want to face or digest. Therefore, it's important to elicit material from its hiding place in your body. Thoughts, memories, and images that you haven't wanted to deal with since childhood exist on a cellular level. The following exercise will help you familiarize yourself with the anger your body may be holding.

EXERCISE: Body Meditation

Get comfortable, clear your mind, take a few deep breaths, and on the exhale, release any negativity or stress you're holding. Gently ask your body about the source of its anger.

1. Beginning at the top of your head, slowly travel through your body, observing places you hold resentment, anger, jealousy, irritation, or annoyance.

2. As you attend to your eyes, jaw, neck, upper back and shoulders, hands, heart, belly, lower back, pelvis, legs, and feet, ask each part about your anger. Wait patiently for your body to respond with a memory, an image, a word, or a phrase. Some parts of the body will say, "No anger here," and others may have a conversation with you, giving you information about your anger's roots. Move from one part to the next.

3. Finish by thanking your body. Take a minute to relax before getting up and moving around. Write the information you received in your anger journal.

If after doing this exercise you cannot identify a source of anger, don't give up. You may receive information about its origins in the next section on movement.

Moving Your Body to Uncover the Source

With movement, anger loses its power and you'll start to change. The changes may be subtle at first. Tight jaws loosen, grinding teeth grind to a halt, shoulders drop down, and frozen pelvises rock back and forth. When the source of your anger is identified and released from tight, contracted muscles, the body regains its natural state.

Fast-paced, assertive movement works best to open muscular blocks and retrieve forgotten material. Energy-freeing exercises may seem silly at first as they involve punching the air with your fists, kicking, jumping, stamping your feet, or running in place. Movement helped Mary face her anger's roots.

When Mary began using movement and energy techniques— standing with her feet shoulder width apart, punching down toward the floor with her fists, and saying the word "no"—something freed up inside of her. As soon as she began to kick, as if to push someone away, she recalled her mother locking her in a dark closet to punish her. This horrific and unpleasant memory shook her to the core. Now she understood the panic attacks she experienced in enclosed spaces and the rage she felt when emotionally cornered.

EXERCISE: Body Movement

Do these exercises a few minutes daily. Each time you do them, you may retrieve more information. They will help you uncover the source and free up energy from stuck places in your body. If you have physical issues or don't often exercise, ask your doctor if you may engage in them.

1. *Start with a Stretch:* Move your head toward your right shoulder and hold it down with your right hand for a few seconds, feeling the stretch. Reverse and do the same on the left. Drop your head and chin forward toward your chest. Then bring your chin up toward the ceiling so that your head falls back. Bring your head back to center. Make circles with your shoulders, forward and backward seven times. Put your hands on your waist and lean backward to stretch your back. Then fall forward, allowing your head and neck to drop down toward the floor. Slowly come back to a standing position.

2. *Moving Arms:* Sitting or standing, with feet shoulder width apart and knees bent slightly, make fists. Punch the air with your fists, fast and

hard, for a complete minute. At the same time, whisper, shout, or think, "Get away." If you do this exercise sitting, press your sit bones into the chair to ground your energy while you punch.

3. *Moving Legs:* With your feet shoulder width apart, stand or sit with your knees bent. Kick forward with each foot, heel first. Kick as fast as you can for a complete minute while whispering, shouting, or thinking, "Get away."

4. *Moving Pelvis:* With your feet shoulder width apart, knees bent slightly and hands on your hips, move your pelvis. Pull it back toward the wall behind you, then quickly slide it forward toward the wall in front of you. Do this movement for a complete minute whispering, shouting, or thinking, "No."

Now write in your journal about the source of your anger, even though you weren't consciously thinking about it while moving. Don't overthink or try to be rational. Write whatever comes to mind, giving your thoughts free range. The information your body holds may surprise you.

Uncovering Irrational Beliefs

Irrational beliefs, not based on facts, may be at the root of your anger. These beliefs pass through your mind quickly, so that if you don't pay attention, you won't know you had them. For instance, the belief, "I'm right and you're wrong" is irrational if you hold on to it stubbornly and refuse to consider conflicting information. If you need to be right, you were likely raised by adults who told you that you were wrong, didn't listen to you, and punished you unfairly. Your anger spikes when someone does not take you seriously or has a different opinion than your own.

The irrational belief "I am unlovable" may occur if you were deprived of love, touch, or nurturance as a child. You probably grew up asking yourself, *What's wrong with me?* Therefore, anger will occur if someone forgets to acknowledge your birthday, return a favor, or ignores you. Here's what happened to Edith, whose belief "I am owed" fed her anger:

Suffering from bouts of bulimia, an eating disorder that involves binge eating followed by throwing up, Edith thought that journaling might help get to the root of what was bothering her. She found herself writing, "They owe me." Now, she remembered both of her parents judging her severely, calling her fat. By spitting out food (in many cultures food is a symbol of love and spitting is a sign of disgust), she expressed anger toward herself for not being the child they wanted and toward them for not giving her the love she believed she deserved. Joining a gym with a punching bag helped her release anger and recognize she could take care of herself.

EXERCISE: Identifying My Irrational Beliefs

Some irrational beliefs are listed below. Write those that you hold or have held in the past in your anger journal. If you hold some not listed here, write them in your journal as well. Knowing these beliefs feed your anger, write a sentence challenging the truthfulness of each belief. Here's an example:

Belief: *I don't fit in anywhere.*

Challenging Idea: *I need to give people a chance so that I can find friends.*

Irrational Beliefs

I don't deserve to be alive.

I don't fit in anywhere.

Nothing will ever work out for me.

Life is drudgery and then you die.

I am special.

Anger is a bad emotion.

I can't trust anyone.

I know what's best, so why should I listen to you?

I must act like I have it together even when I don't.

It's not safe to let anyone know my business.

I was born to please other people and make them happy.

I'm right and you're wrong.

Because irrational beliefs have power over our psyches, they feed our anger. Now that you have identified yours and challenged them, look to see what pictures your mind may be holding on to.

Images at the Root of Toxic Anger

Images that appear in dreams, doodles, and drawings can lead you back to the source of your anger. Mikala used an image to free herself from irrational anger.

After one or two dates, Mikala stopped calling the women to whom she felt most attracted. She joined a personal growth group in hopes of changing her behavior. A woman in the group wore bright red lipstick. When Mikala looked at her, she felt angry. The next day she set up an easel in her apartment and did several paintings of the woman's red lips. Then she remembered her mother kissing her goodbye with red painted lips before she went out dancing. The image helped her discover unresolved anger toward her mother for leaving her alone many nights. She now understood the role feeling rejected played in her life. Two years later, she was in a committed relationship.

You too may be drawn to an image that can provide information about the birth of your angry self. Try to remember repetitive dreams, such as being locked in a room with no escape, or daydreams in which you, like David, overcame Goliath. Visualize the nose or eyes or an article of clothing of a person you despise. Draw pictures of the images that come to mind in your journal to help you bring unconscious material to consciousness.

Modeling Your Perpetrator's Behavior

Some of you follow in your perpetrators' footsteps; your anger looks like theirs. This is not purposeful behavior on your part. It's the last thing you want. But it may lead you to the source of your anger.

Copying the actions of people who treated you poorly in the past is called *introjection*. You take on their voices, postures, and behaviors in an attempt to gain control and make their anger less frightening and upsetting. This process backfires because you lose a connection to your true self. Here's what Janiya realized when she started an argument with Dashawn, her boyfriend:

> *Janiya sarcastically asked Dashawn why he would attend a dinner at his former place of work, telling him that he would be wasting his time. Actually, she didn't have a problem with his going but enjoyed making him feel bad about it. When she looked at her behavior, she remembered her mother doing the same thing to her. If she was looking forward to a school trip, her mother found some way to squash her joy. Never having confronted her mother, she became a spoiler like her mother.*

Think about a time when you behaved like someone whose actions you found upsetting or like someone you abhorred. When you observed yourself acting or sounding like that person, did you feel ashamed, angry with yourself, or sad that you had copied this behavior? This behavior may be emerging from your unconscious. In your anger journal, describe exactly what happened in the past: who, when, and where.

Remembering Before Conscious Memory

You may have to go back to the womb to find the source of your anger. Even though you won't remember that experience, you have a felt sense about it within you. According to epigenetics, stressors, both internal and external, experienced by your mother cause changes in your fetal genes, changing the behavior of the person who you become (Lipton 2005, Wilner 2020). A mother's experiences during pregnancy such as war, food scarcity, smoking, taking drugs, arguing, physical violence, and shouting can change her baby's ability to handle anger after birth.

But having a bad experience in the womb does not need to scar you for life. By making every effort to uncover the source of your anger, accept it, and transform it, you are helping your genes repair themselves and return to their natural state.

EXERCISE: Visualizing Womb Exercise

Sit comfortably and take slow deep breaths. Relaxing deeply, imagine yourself as a fetus floating in a cold, hostile womb. Perhaps your mother does not have enough food, has taken medicine that disagrees with her, or is being abused by her partner. Imagine or sense how your fetal body feels. Allow and witness whatever arises, then describe this experience in your journal. Now give yourself a big hug to erase feelings left from the cold womb.

Connect the Present to the Past

Current situations that trigger your anger, no matter how infuriating, afford you the opportunity to uncover its source. According to Carl Jung's theory of synchronicity, events and people in the present are strategically placed to remind you of something from the past. A current event may cause you to remember painful experiences that happened before you knew how to defend yourself, giving you the opportunity to heal the past. Here's what Kelly remembered.

Kelly couldn't relate to her mother-in-law. Every word that came out of the woman's mouth irritated her. Yet she didn't understand why; her mother-in-law was polite, intelligent, and treated her well. During a kicking exercise in an energy class, she realized that her mother-in-law resembled her older sister, Samantha. She had been jealous of beautiful, athletic Samantha growing up. Could she be jealous of her mother-in-law? After sharing this theory with friends, she felt unburdened and invited her mother-in-law to lunch.

Think about a person who currently triggers your anger or a situation that incites it and ask yourself the following questions:

- Who in my past does this person remind me of?

- What situations in the past am I reminded of?

- Did something like this occur during my adolescence, childhood, or infancy?

- Could something like this have happened in school, at church, on the playground, or in a car?

If memories are missing or you were too young to remember, ask older siblings, cousins, parents, friends of the family, or caretakers what may have occurred. Or you can put your imagination to work and make them up. A made-up answer is a good way to retrieve hidden material tucked away in the unconscious. The stories you create will hold some grain of truth.

EXERCISE: Empty Chair

One final method to help you get to the source of your anger involves having a heart-to-heart conversation with your angry self.

Sit in a chair facing an empty chair. The empty chair represents your angry self. Ask that self, "How did you come to exist?" Now, sit in that chair and respond, sharing what you know about your anger's origins. When you finish, switch seats again and thank your angry self for providing this information. If you feel uncomfortable speaking out loud, do the exercise quietly in your head or write the dialogue between these two parts in your anger journal.

Even if you don't want to blame someone else for your anger, remember that when you were a child, you had little control over what happened to you. Some bad things may have occurred that resulted in your present-day anger. It is important to bring those memories into consciousness instead of repressing them. Through understanding, acceptance, and forgiveness, you can deal with the events that occurred in those years when your brain was still forming.

Deeply Felt, Old Anger Can Heal

You hide the information that you don't want to know about yourself in your body, and this is particularly true of anger. You may resist owning your anger because you want others to view you positively. If you were raised to believe that anger is bad, you don't want to acknowledge that mean thoughts enter your mind or you sometimes have a desire to hurt another person or you have fantasies of revenge. By masking your anger, you cover an infection with a bandage without getting rid of the underlying bacteria that can make you sick. Since each of us bears responsibility for our anger, to some degree, because it's our limbic system and our brain that reacts to triggering events in a toxic manner, it's up to us to find the roots of our anger and change our behavior.

This step helps uncover the root of your anger and bring it into consciousness. Tools and approaches used included identifying irrational beliefs, journaling, meditation, movement, asking questions about the past, drawing and painting, identifying negative self-talk, and releasing blocked energy from muscles in your body. The next step will help you actively deal with your anger by grounding it, thereby creating safety for yourself and those around you.

Ground: Become an Anger Lightning Rod

The more a person can feel contact with the ground...the more she can handle a broader spectrum of feelings.

—Jerry Nabb, *Core Energetic Concepts of Grounding*

Anja reacted to the car that abruptly pulled out in front of her and almost caused an accident. Heart pumping fast and adrenaline surging through her body, she pressed down hard on the gas pedal. She caught up at the next light and prepared to get out to tell this person off. Though she was ready for a fight and full of vigor, thoughts of her recent promise to her family to maintain control kept her in the car. After seeing it was a young girl, she congratulated herself for maintaining her composure.

Like lightning, Anja's anger came on suddenly, out of nowhere. If you had asked what she felt a second earlier, she would have said relaxed. Her anger was intense, not a mild irritation that could be shoved aside, but a strong push to get even. Every muscle tightened, her teeth clamped down, and energy shot out of her pupils. Like lightning, she needed to release this energy. She wanted to grab the other driver and shake her.

If Anja knew how to ground her energy, she could have become a lightning rod to bring her anger to earth and keep her impulsive behavior at bay. Grounding exercises allow you to maintain control, and if you ride a horse called "anger"—and we all have that animal in our stables—you will hold the reins.

Balancing Your Energy

Grounding involves body movements and exercises that balance your energy flow so that it moves down away from your head toward your legs and feet (Lowen and Lowen 1977; Nabb 1999). With toxic anger, your energy enters a state of imbalance, rising upward into the chest, shoulders, upper back, neck, and head. This upward displacement leads to sweating, itching, panting, screaming, yelling, aching heads, burning sensations, throwing things, grinding teeth, ruminating, negative thinking, and losing control. Simultaneously, energy in your lower body decreases, so that your, pelvis, legs, and feet, the parts that anchor you and keep you in reality, lose energy. Grounding reverses this process, bringing the energy back toward the ground where it belongs, restoring the natural distribution, so that no one muscle group or organ suffers from having too much or too little.

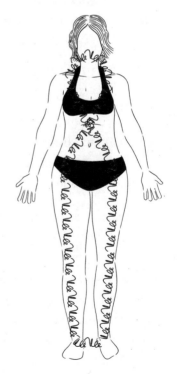

When you think of being grounded, visualize your energy streaming down from the north pole (your head) to the south pole (your feet) and back up again. This continuous flow energizes your physiological system at the same time as it pacifies your nervous system. The energy moves in a figure eight: up one side of your body from your feet, crossing in the middle at the solar plexus, and continuing up the opposite side (Reich 1972). It crosses over at the roof of your mouth (the soft palate) and returns to your feet.

Grounding means being in reality, taking responsibility, staying present, and maintaining a relaxed and natural physical state. It helps you deal with strong emotions so that when grounded,

Healthy Energy Flow

you can talk about your anger in a reasonable way. Grounding exercises help you breathe freely and handle difficult situations with relative ease. You'll cope with stress, feel safe and secure in your body, decrease your anger, and use problem-solving techniques to achieve positive results. Your awareness sharpens, and feelings integrate with thoughts so that they work together as one.

Grounding techniques also decrease physical arousal. When angry, your brain sends signals to release stress-related chemicals into your body that prepare you to fight or flee and move your blood to areas that will allow you to react quickly and instinctively to save yourself. This process fires up your nervous system, bringing about physiological arousal, which would make sense if you were living among dangerous animals. But because you live in a community with other people, an overly excited nervous system makes your anger dangerous. You could catch on fire and explode in anger, or if you suppress anger, the hormones associated with it may poison your insides and instigate health issues.

Grounding Supports Your Health

When toxic anger rises upward in your body, it brings intense, fiery energy into vulnerable organs such as the heart, lungs, and brain. Your muscles contract, holding on to adrenaline, neuro-adrenaline, cortisol, and testosterone, which causes your blood pressure to rise. This occurred for Nadine when she forgot to ground her anger.

> *Nadine, a yoga therapist, raged at her fiancé for changing the dates of their vacation without consulting her. She grabbed a tennis racket and beat the mattress. Later that night, an intense and painful headache woke her. Her blood pressure had skyrocketed. Expressive work such as hitting, kicking, and yelling is not an option when you're on fire. You are ripe to hurt yourself—envision an asthma attack, a nasty argument, or cutting yourself cooking—or someone else. Nadine did not take the time to ground before hitting the mattress, so she inflicted harm upon her body.*

Grounding exercises should both precede and follow the release of strong emotion. They ensure that energy flows downward and that the fire goes out. The overall lesson for Nadine—and one that we all need to learn—is that anger has to be respected. Do grounding exercises before and after you release anger, even before you talk about it. As soon as you experience heat or arousal moving up in your body, pause, ground, feel your feet, and allow your anger to dissipate. Following are three gentle grounding exercises Nadine used to restore her sense of peace.

Stretch Between Heaven and Earth

Stand or sit with your back straight, feet shoulder width apart, and toes pointing straight ahead. Reach both arms up toward the sky, stretching your upper body. At the same time, press your feet hard into the ground without locking your knees. Experience a lengthening in the middle of your body where heaven and earth meet. Hold for thirty seconds.

Comparison Walk

Walk around the room on your tiptoes with your neck and head slanted to one side. Note how you feel in this ungrounded position? Now walk "grounded," with your neck straight, knees slightly bent, feet fully on the floor, spine straight, eyes open and in contact with the objects in the room. Experience the difference.

Foot Massage

Take off your shoes and wiggle your toes. Massage each foot, sole, top, instep, ball, toes, and heel, for three minutes. Then hold each foot gently in the palm of your hand. If you can't reach your feet, ask someone to massage them for you. Or rub the soles and sides of your feet, toes bent under, against the floor, stimulating them through your movements.

Connecting to the earth through these simple exercises provides safety and stability. Whereas toxic anger endangers health, grounding enables you to make good choices for yourself and others.

Grounding Means Standing Up for Yourself

Theoretically, the sky represents big ideas and spirituality, and the earth represents being in reality, pragmatic, and responsible. You're able to deal with facts rather than living in fantasy or harboring illusions under the influence of strong anger. Being grounded means that you make good decisions and keep your mind oriented in the present rather than the past or future.

Standing represents maturity whereas lying down is associated with regression, infancy, and dependence (Pierrakos 1995). This concept is extremely important for women who have been dependent on men financially and emotionally. When husbands left their wives for younger women in the past, the wives—our mothers, grandmothers, and aunts—didn't have the means or knowledge to stand up for themselves. Often, their standard of living fell, sometimes to the poverty line. In the following example, Amy stood up for herself, using grounding to turn her life around.

After fifteen years of marriage, Amy's ex-husband left, revealing he was gay. He also manipulated the legal system to keep her from receiving alimony. Amy was overcome with sadness and rage. Completing grounding exercises first thing in the morning and last thing before bed, and at any time she began to argue with him in her mind's eye, helped Amy calm down, stand on her own two feet, and accept the situation. Feeling stronger, she emanated confidence and was promoted to a highly coveted position in her company. Years later, when tragedy hit again—the unexpected passing of her brother, her son's cancer diagnosis, and her mother's debilitating stroke, all within a year's time—she turned to the same exercises. Grounding helped her remain strong and gave her the courage to deal with the anger attached to feelings of helplessness.

To facilitate your ability to face hardships without panicking, lashing out, or becoming bitter, do the following grounding exercises daily. They will help you feel confident, strong, safe, and secure. They will bring your anger down to earth. During these exercises, energy may release from your muscles, causing your body to shake or vibrate. This is normal. If you have health concerns, ask your doctor if they are appropriate for you.

Four of my favorite grounding exercises follow. The bow integrates the head, heart, and pelvis at the same time as it grounds your energy; the waterfall brings energy away from the head; squatting and jumping brings your energy to the earth quickly; and hugging a tree connects you to your roots (Lowen and Lowen 1977; Wilner and Black 2009).

The Bow

Place your feet shoulder width apart and point your toes forward. Make fists with your hands and place them at the small of your back. Bend your knees and roll your pelvis toward the wall in front of you. At the same time, roll your shoulders back so that you arch your back and push out your chest. Point your chin down toward your chest and raise your eyes up toward the ceiling. Work up to staying in this position, although it may feel uncomfortable, for two minutes. Trembling means that your energy is releasing and flowing into your entire body.

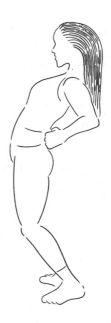

The Bow Grounding Exercise

The Roll-Over/Waterfall

Stand with your feet shoulder width apart and slightly pigeon-toed. Pointing your toes in engages the muscles that run up the sides of your legs. Bend your knees slightly and roll over from the waist till your fingers touch the floor and the top of your head faces the ground. Relax into the stretch, paying attention to your breath. Extend your tailbone up toward the ceiling. Now, straighten your legs slightly and feel the stretch in your

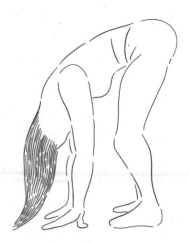

The Waterfall Grounding Exercise

hamstrings. Remain in this position two minutes. Roll up to standing, slowly, one vertebra at a time. If you do this exercise sitting, push your feet hard into the floor and your sit bones into the chair.

Half-Squat Grounding (Alternative to Roll-Over/Waterfall)

The half-squat grounding exercise is designed for people with back problems and those who cannot bend over. To move energy away from your head and pelvis, stand with your feet shoulder width apart and knees bent in a squat position. Push your feet hard against the floor and return to a straight-legged position, feeling a stretch in your calves. Do this movement quickly, approximately twenty to forty times. You will notice energy flowing in your legs and feet.

Squatting and Jumping

(Do this exercise if you're physically fit or have your doctor's permission.)

Squat as low as possible with your feet a little wider than your shoulders. Jump up and down five times, each time returning to the original squat position. As you do this exercise, concentrate on bringing your energy down and away from your upper body to the floor.

Hugging a Tree

Next time you're in nature, pick a tree. It can be old and gnarled or young and sprightly. Stand close to it and press your feet into the earth, bending your knees slightly. Then touch the tree with both hands or wrap your arms around it. With eyes closed, receive its energy.

Grounding exercises like these support taking responsibility, logical thinking, and problem solving.

Grounding Your Thinking

Toxic anger, whether suppressed, expressed, or passive-aggressive, represents the inverse of logical thought. Fed by arousal and emotion, it feeds on blame, low self-esteem, finger-pointing, perceiving others at fault, and desiring to punish them. Because grounding exercises carry excess energy away from the head, they help restore rational thinking. For example, Victoria needed to ground in order to make a good decision.

Victoria's live-in boyfriend cheated, called her weak and spineless, refused sex with her, ignored her birthday, and stole money from her wallet. Every cell in her brain said, End it and leave him. *But frozen, like an iceberg, she feared making a decision she would regret. Thoughts like* Maybe he'll change, I am imagining it's worse than it is, *and* I won't meet anyone better *flooded her mind. Raised by an ultrastrong single mother, Victoria knew how to submit, give in, and give up, but she had never made her own decisions or taken responsibility for her life. Daily grounding helped her view herself as a strong person. Soon she told Robert, "It's over," packed her bags, and left the apartment for good.*

Victoria enjoyed the following two grounding exercises. Try them for yourself.

The Ostrich

Stand with your knees softly bent and your feet shoulder width apart. Place your weight on your right foot and bend your right knee as much as possible. At the same time, use the big toe of your left foot for balance without putting weight on your left foot. Stay in this position for one minute, then switch legs. Place your weight on your left foot and bend your left knee. Use your right toe to balance yourself without placing weight on the right foot. Hold this position for one moment before relaxing and letting go.

The Heel Stamp

Stand or sit with your feet shoulder width apart and your knees flexed. Loosen your jaw and allow your shoulders to drop down. Rise up on the balls of your feet and then immediately stomp down hard with your heels. Do this twenty times, moving quickly. Now add fists. Punch down with your fists toward the floor, at the same time you stomp with your heels, and loudly vocalize "no" or "my way."

Grounding exercises help you integrate practical, problem-solving thoughts into your personal life.

Grounding Enhances Your Senses

There's a relationship between grounding and your senses. My students, after engaging in weekly grounding exercises, found that grounding improved their sensory experience: their eyes could see, ears could hear, hands could touch, voices could speak the truth, and feet could contact the earth (Wilner 2012). There is truth to this. When you're grounded you listen and hear the other person's point of view. You don't leap ahead and think about what to say next. Your gaze softens and you receive the other person, whereas when you're angry you look out of narrow, contracted eyelids and pupils that cut the other down to size. Because energy gets blocked in the eyes, especially if you have experienced trauma or have seen things you didn't want to see, do the following eye movement exercise to release tension and improve your grounding.

EXERCISE: Draw a Square with Your Eyes

Keep your head and neck still and breathe normally. Make a square with your eye movements: start by moving your pupils from the far left to the far right, then move them from up to down, from far right to far left, and finally from down to up. Do this five times. Now, reverse the movement, moving your pupils from far right to far left five times. When eye blocks release, negative emotions may emerge, or you may feel refreshed and energized. Take a minute to observe your feelings and then describe them in your journal. Do this exercise three times per week followed by the waterfall to ground your energy.

EXERCISE: Describe Your Grounding Questions

Here are some questions about your current state of grounding. If you're learning about grounding for the first time or hearing it presented in a different way, it's good to ask in what areas of your life you could be more grounded. In your journal, answer the following questions about grounding in your life:

1. List three aspects of your life in which you are ungrounded. Examples: Can't balance checkbook. Scream at children when they don't pick up after themselves. Forget to take car in for inspection.

2. If there were one major life experience in your past that ungrounded you, what would it be? Examples: Parents divorcing. Being held back in school. Bullying on the playground.

3. List three actions that help you ground when you feel angry. Examples: Call a friend. Push hard against a wall. Hug a tree.

4. Describe how your anger changes when you are grounded. Examples: Breathing normalizes. Able to talk about it. Find a solution.

Physical Signs of Grounding

You can learn a lot about grounding by observing your legs and feet. Legs and feet indicate whether you take responsibility for yourself or give in to someone else's will, stand up or fall down, move forward in life, and deal with emotions positively. The following information comes from my studies of body reading and my work with chakras (Brennan 1988; Pierrakos 1987). The twelve chakras are points at which vital energy from the universe enters the body according to Eastern theory.

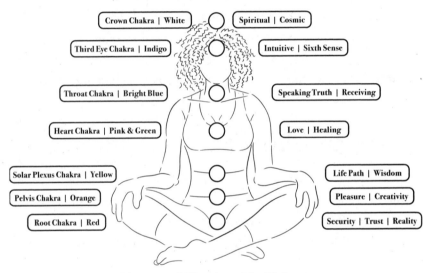

Placement & Meaning of the Chakras

When your energy flows well at an entry point, the behavior linked to that chakra is life enhancing. When the energy at the entry point is blocked or diminished, a problem exists. The legs and feet are associated specifically with the first four chakras: root, pelvis, solar plexus, and heart.

- Firmly planted feet represent the root chakra, safety and security. A shaky stance, such as moving back and forth from one foot to the other, or putting all your weight on one foot, indicates insecurity.

- When grounded, the four corners of each foot (excluding the toes) touch the floor. The soles of your feet press into the earth with your weight centered in the middle of your foot. Improve your grounding by pointing your feet straight ahead when you walk.

- Toes curling under and toes that lift away from the ground signify feeling unsafe. Visualize your toes relaxing and straightening out. Stretch your toes to create space between them.

- Ultra-high arches occur when muscles in the center of the foot contract. They can unground you. To help your arches relax, roll your feet over a soft tennis ball.

- Collapsed arches or flat feet reflect a tendency to give in to others or give up. To rectify, wear arch supports in your shoes. When walking barefoot, roll to the sides of your feet to give yourself an arch.

- Ankles represent the relationship between your life force (second chakra/pelvis, the pleasure center) and the earth. If you wish for more pleasure or vitality, massage your ankles, wear ankle bracelets, and dress in orange, the color of the second chakra.

- Ankles, calves, knees, and thighs that roll in toward each other (pronate inward) reflect feeling unsafe and a tendency to give in or fall down. Change your stance. Roll these body parts away from each other. Stand in this new position for a minute or two each day.

- Sprained, injured, or broken ankles or legs signify a lack of grounding. You may be responding to a situation with toxic anger, suppressed or impulsive. The more frequently you practice grounding exercises, the less likely you are to get hurt.

- Calves represent the third chakra, the solar plexus, and your life path. Energy flowing through them indicates that you're in touch with your feelings and happy about your chosen path.

Tense calves reflect blocked energy and difficulty processing emotions. Massage your calves to free up your energy. Also, stimulate the muscles by lying on a mat and kicking sixty to one hundred times, raising each leg three inches from the mat.

- Knees represent the fourth chakra, the heart. Keeping them slightly bent will protect the joints. You will feel more connected to the earth and to your heart.

- Calves rotating away from your body, such as in a bow-legged stance, mean that the energy disperses before it reaches the ground. To improve grounding, stand with your legs three to six inches apart. Do this for two or three minutes a day to establish a new body habit.

- Locked knees (legs ramrod straight) send energy up toward your head, keeping you ungrounded. They enable toxic anger. Bend your knees slightly so that energy moves through the knee joints into your lower legs and feet.

- Because the thighs connect to the hips, pelvis, and root chakra, they bring sexual energy (your life force) to the ground. Massage or tap your thighs to invigorate them.

- Variations in skin color, texture, or the temperature of the legs and feet indicate energy blocks. Look for birthmarks, hot or cold skin, and changes in skin color. When you find a block, run in place or kick lying on a mat for a full minute, as fast as you can, to help release stuck energy.

Being attentive to your legs and feet helps you integrate earth into your life.

Meeting Mother Earth

Of course, grounding concerns the earth. In American Indian traditions, Mother Earth represents a sense of oneness with the planet. We are interdependent with the earth, which sustains life through its resources, embodying a nurturing presence. This image carries over to the nurturing you received as an infant and the care that you provide your own children. Energy theorists, child psychologists, and pediatricians (Karp 2015; Mahler, Pine, and Bergman 2000; Pierrakos 1987) tell us that when babies and children are held, loved, and fed, the energy they receive grounds them. The main nurturer, usually the mother— although others including fathers and grandparents take on this role— is responsible for providing security because infants can't ground themselves. When held close to the chest, hearing the heartbeat, and taking in the odor of love, infants feel safe. This establishes a strong attachment. If you lacked positive nurturing experiences, the following grounding exercise may help you heal.

EXERCISE: With a Mother's Eyes

Hold a small pillow close to your chest. Look at the pillow and visualize yourself as a baby. Allow loving energy to flow from your eyes, arms, hands, and heart into the pillow. Envision welcoming your infant and experience a sense of oneness. Sense your feelings as you hold this pose for a full minute.

Nurturing is as important as air and water, and mental health problems can begin during infancy when babies don't receive physical touch. Some of these adverse effects can be reversed through grounding.

Safe Baby Questions

- Think about the person who mothered or nurtured you during your first few years of life. (A) What made you feel safe? (B) What made you feel unsafe? Write the answers in your journal.

- Then think about people in your current life. (A) What do they do to make you feel safe? (B) What do they do to make you feel unsafe? (C) What do you do to make them feel safe? (D) What do you do that makes them feel unsafe?

Write the answers in your journal.

Releasing Anger into the Earth

Whether you have Anger-Out, Anger-In, or Passive-Aggressive anger, grounding helps your anger change its form and consequences. By turning it over to the earth, negative vibrations, ugly words, and noxious chemicals reduce so they can no longer harm your body or your relationships. The next step, *Release*, builds on grounding so that your anger disperses in a positive form. Toxic anger transforms when it's no longer hidden and locked away in your unconscious. It can then flow harmlessly and harmoniously through your body without affecting those in your immediate environment. Releasing anger will change its energy from heavy and dark to lighter and brighter.

Release: Name It, Claim It, Let It Go, Let It Flow

The beast within
Though small in size
Has the strength of giants
And fiery eyes.

—Anonymous, The Beast Within

Danita's father, a famous novelist, hit her mother in the stomach while she was pregnant with Danita. He continued to abuse her mother and have affairs with other women throughout her childhood. Disgusted with him, Danita took steps to save herself, even if her mother wouldn't. She moved out of their home, found a job, and signed up for body awareness classes. Energy exercises helped her release the hatred and anger that had built up over the years. Her body felt lighter, free, and cleansed. Eventually, she wrote a memoir focusing on domestic violence and as she wrote, she continued to heal.

Letting go of toxic anger means letting go of the beast that feeds it. It requires you to release your negative thoughts, the masks you wear to hide your anger from yourself and others, and the energy blocked in tight muscles.

Reasons to Release Negative Thinking

Fear-based, angry thinking is detrimental to your health and ability to experience pleasure. Anxious thoughts reflect your concern about successfully handling future events, and resentful ones occur when you consider situations unfair and unjust. Both tell your brain to spew out chemicals that cause disease and mental confusion.

Your anxiety- and fear-based, angry thinking drives you to choose safety over fulfillment so that you're more likely to say "no" rather than "yes" to opportunities that present themselves. Perhaps you didn't study a subject you felt passionate about because someone said, "You will never find a job in that field." Fear intrudes on success, telling you to put on the brakes, but eventually you may resent moments that you missed. Combined with anger, Rhonda's fear-based thinking began to affect her sleep:

> *Rhonda, age forty, had recently been waking up three to five times a night. She wondered if her sleep issues could be due to stress— she was suing her previous employer for gender discrimination and her case would soon be heard. Anger about the unfair treatment she received mixed with her fear about losing in court, and feeling humiliated if she were to lose. She couldn't help but wonder if she had made a mistake. Maybe she shouldn't have sued in the first place. She couldn't stop questioning herself.*

Negative thoughts toward others are often fueled by hurt, excitement, or both. You harbor dark thoughts that energize you and entertain visions of punishing others for what you believe they did to you. You feel adverse excitement as you chase down the highway after the red sports car that was riding your tail. Or you come alive when you complain, blame, or judge those closest to you—your spouse, parents, and friends. Negativity can animate you and keep your anger at a heightened level. However, the negative excitement you derive when thinking about getting even is bad for your body and for your relationships—negative excitement differs from the pleasure associated with positive excitement. Here's what happened to Laurie:

Laurie's anger toward the opposite sex made her feel strong. Both her high school boyfriend and her ex-husband betrayed her with other women. When she caught her current boyfriend watching porn, she lashed out verbally, slapped him, and broke a window. A neighbor summoned the police. Forced to attend anger management classes, she admitted to the other participants that she found anger exciting. In the class, she learned to value peace.

If you enjoy the sensation of anger surging through you and take adverse pleasure in negative thinking and the arousal that follows it, you may fail to see how it's hurting you. Perhaps in the moment, you feel strong, thinking, *I'm not going to take it anymore.* For the few seconds, minutes, or hours that anger feels good, it blocks out the feelings that accompany it—fear, grief, hurt, pain, and shame. Feeling excited by its intensity, you fail to see how it interferes with your ability to think clearly and your intention to live a calmer, happier life. Consider Mildred's situation:

Speaking quickly and erratically, eyes flashing with excitement, Mildred retold the story of escaping from a war zone. She described her uncle lying bloody on the floor and her family's escape over the mountains, running for their lives. She expressed hatred toward the enemy, keeping her anger alive and keeping the underlying pain and terror at bay. Even though her friends felt compassion for her, hearing this story repeatedly upset them. When they talked to Mildred about it, she recognized that she needed to release her fear and anger and deal with the underlying trauma. Only then could she create a new story.

Although it's important to acknowledge angry feelings and not lock them away in the muscles of your body, once they're acknowledged and shared, you need to let them go. You would not hold on to a live grenade, and neither should you hold on to a toxic emotional state. I dealt with this myself when John C. Pierrakos, my mentor in the field of somatic therapy, challenged me to release my toxic anger:

He said, "You have a killer inside you." At first, I denied it. "I am sweet, nice, and empathetic. I care about people. Who, me, a killer? Killer Miller?" (Miller was my maiden name.) But then I had to admit that I do have a dark side that's intense. Some of it's due to biology and human nature, some I inherited, and some comes from my personality and life experiences. Using energy, movement, and meditation techniques, I began the process of unblocking my energy and releasing the hurt, pain, and anger that I carried since early childhood—some of which I had suppressed.

Negative Thoughts You Need to Release

This section presents the types of negative thoughts that lead to toxic anger. Some of them were addressed in chapter 1. You need to bring these thoughts into conscious awareness so that you can release them and let them go.

Overreactions

You make situations much worse than they are. You make them bigger and more dangerous, creating fear and anger in your body. Here are some examples of overreactions:

- *My girlfriend says she is taking a class and then going out with her friends. I don't believe her. This could be the end. I may just end it with her first.*

- *My landlord doesn't want to renew my lease because I made a complaint. I think he is going to kick me out and I have no place to go. I will be homeless.*

- *I don't like the way I performed on my last job. I should have done better. I am angry at myself. I want to hurt myself. I am a complete failure. I will never be good at anything. I should just die.*

- *My wife had an affair. I can't forgive her. If people find out, they will think less of me. She has trashed our family and the values we hold. I want to hurt her and I want to kill the guy.*

- *Two days after the job interview, they called and left a message asking to speak again. I guess I didn't get it or they would have said so. I am so bummed.*

Habitual, Automatic, and Subliminal Thoughts

Consider the number of thoughts you have that begin with "I can't," "I should," "It's a waste of my time," and "They don't love me, or they would have…" Negative thoughts come in the form of a whisper that you learn to tune out over time, or they're automatic, like brushing your teeth, so you stop paying attention to them. They can live beneath conscious awareness, keeping you in the dark about the number you have on any given day. But they're there, and they can poison your mind. Sometimes these thoughts arise automatically. Imagine standing in line to buy tickets and the movie is about to start. You are impatient with the cashier and *What's her problem?!* crosses your mind. This thought, laced with anger, arises out of the blue.

Obsessive Thoughts, Ruminations, Repetitive Thinking

These occur when your mind gets caught on one thought, repeating it over and over. It's particularly stressful when you can't get your brain to stop. It might involve thinking you will set the house on fire, make a mistake, or change the mind of a suitor who rejected you. For instance, whenever Jerri was alone at night, the threat of a break-in kept her up all night. Even with several locks and a chair in front of the door, she couldn't stop this thought from cycling through her mind.

Lack of Fairness

You want life to be fair, and when you discover it isn't, anger results. If you're married, you keep track of who does more housework or child-care. At work, you do the same with colleagues. Then you struggle to suppress your anger, or you stoop to making hurtful or sarcastic comments.

Negative Beliefs

Beliefs about yourself or others that you accept as true can feed your anger. They're passed down through families or they grow out of your early experiences. Denise, who grew up with two workaholic, college professor parents who rarely lifted their heads out of their books, felt neglected. Her go-to belief was *I am owed*. It colored her life and transferred onto others. When she didn't get exactly what she wanted from them, she would be overcome with anger and plot to get them back.

Prejudices, Stereotypes, and Preconceived Notions About Groups of People

You think negatively about those who differ from you in some way (skin color, race, ethnicity, gender, religion, education, social class, disability). This irrational thinking results from deep fears and insecurities. We all need to look deep inside to identify well-hidden prejudices. Regarding her struggle with this, a professor shared,

> I attended a meeting about racism and sexism in the educational system. A colleague brought up the number of trans students in our classes. When I used the pronoun "she" instead of "they" to describe a student, she drew this to my attention. In response, I shared my anger at having to change my pronouns and make these students special. This incident led me to sign up for diversity classes.

Negative thoughts cloud your ability to experience pleasure. They take up brain space and trigger anger. You even have negative thoughts about your anger, worrying about losing your temper in public or being rejected socially because of your attitude. Additionally, your worries are tinged with anger. Thinking about getting lost while driving, you angrily wish you didn't have to drive alone. Shame and embarrassment often follow the release of anger because some part of you knows anger is not your truth. Toxic anger has taken you away from your authentic self.

The following release exercise will help you let go of negative thoughts, toxic anger, and their adverse effects on your body. Blocked energy will release from your muscles and flow back into your body, becoming one with your life force.

EXERCISE: Releasing Negative Thoughts

This exercise involves moving your body quickly while verbalizing a negative feeling. The bilateral movements, punching and stamping with opposite sides of your body, work with your brain's frontal lobes to help your anger release (Shapiro and Forest 2016).

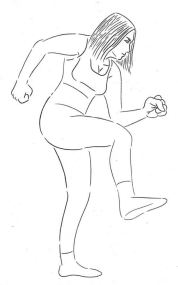

Stamping Exercise to Release Blocked Energy

Choose a safe space to do this exercise that will not create stress for the people or pets you live with.

- Write a negative thought in your journal; it could be an overreaction, a repetitive thought, a criticism, or a judgment. Then say it out loud. For example: "It's your fault the trip was canceled," "I'm angry that no one helps around here," or "Who do you think you are?"

- Then claim the anger underlying your thought with a short statement using one of these words: angry, mad, disappointed, revenge, hate, annoyed, hurt, frustrated, jealous. Example: "I am angry with you," or "I am disappointed in you." Now combine this statement with movement.

- Say the statement over and over, as fast as you can, at the same time as you do one of the following movements: run in place, punch the air in front of you, kick like a karate master, jump up and down, or hit a mattress with fists or a tennis racket. Do this for one or two minutes.

- Finish by grounding. Do a Bow, Waterfall, Ostrich, or Heel Stamp exercise. End by placing your palms on your heart.

Do this exercise once a day for two weeks and then two or three times a week. Soon you will let go of negative thoughts and experience more vitality and life. After the exercise, you may feel relaxed, or if you hold lots of pent-up anger, you may, at first, feel tired or drained. Shame or remorse are natural responses to freeing up anger. Physical signs of release include yawning, sighing, crying, laughing, shaking, twitching, sweating, coughing, burping, yelling, jaw trembling, and teeth chattering. They're normal reactions to letting go of tension.

Because you tend to hide your anger behind a facade, you need to release your anger masks as well—the things you do or say to cover over your anger.

Release Your Negative Masks

You wear masks, like what is worn on Halloween, but these aren't visible. They exist to hide your anger. You don't want to be known as a woman with an anger problem. Although anger masks seem to provide emotional safety, you lose touch with your true self. By obscuring your anger, you fail to expose your authentic feelings, and you can't communicate your anger in a healthy way. For example, when Ruth smiled as she talked about her vicious divorce and unequitable settlement, I found her facial expression unsettling and her message confusing. She explained, "If you can't see my pain, it doesn't hurt as much." The listener is often left confused about whether to trust the words or the facial expression.

Even when your anger is reasonable, rational, and justified, masks stop you from taking a position, problem solving, and repairing relationships. Destiny learned this growing up in her family and promised she would never do the same.

Destiny's family wore the "all is good" mask even when they were hurt or angry. When Mom lost her job due to discrimination, they weren't allowed to express angry feelings or talk about it. Because they didn't discuss or address the problem, Mom didn't get legal counsel, unemployment, or suggestions from friends about where to look for a new job.

Here are some masks women use to conceal their anger.

Blame. In addition to being a type of negative thinking, blame is used to excuse your anger. It says, "I have every right to be angry because of what you did." By accusing another of wrongdoing, in an irritated or demeaning tone of voice, your eyebrows pulling together, and your lips turning downward, you make the statement, "It's your fault, not mine, so my anger is justified." Blame hinders you from taking your share of responsibility, which is often fifty-fifty, and blame covers over authentic emotions. Maria used blame to cover over her grief and the anger that accompanied it.

Contemptuous of Leo, her husband, a successful and widely respected attorney, Maria blamed him for overspending and withholding affection. Never having forgiven her father for dying when she was ten, she directed her anger toward Leo, her only other significant male relationship.

Rationalizations. You make seemingly logical explanations about why you're not angry, even when your body displays signs of anger and stress. Here is an example:

> *Through tight lips, Nadia explained, "We were planning to go to this new restaurant that everyone is talking about. I bought a dress for the occasion. My boyfriend called at the last moment to say his car wouldn't start; it seemed like an engine problem. I told him, "I understand, I'm not angry."*

Nadia doesn't own feeling disappointed, one of anger's sidekicks. Instead, she says, "I understand," trying to appear rational and kind. What she doesn't realize is that it's normal to have more than one feeling; she can be both understanding and disappointed at the same time. If you don't acknowledge or verbalize all of your feelings, those you ignore will find a home in your body; they will be *somaticized*. The word "somaticize" means that when feelings aren't verbalized, they move into your body.

Justifications and explanations. You may use reasonable explanations to mask your anger. For example, during a discussion about the lack of healthy food in a school cafeteria, one of the women digressed to talk about her childhood, saying, "My mother neglected me. She would go out with her friends and forget to feed me. But I understand why she did that; her mother treated her even worse."

The fallacy that this woman operates under is that you can't be angry if people have good reasons for their behavior. Even when this is the case, it's still appropriate to be angry if you experienced hurt, fear, abuse, or disrespect by someone's actions. You can't explain a problem away either. Although a reasonable explanation exists, you still need to own your negative feeling if you have one. Here's what Rebecca experienced:

> *When Rebecca's teenage son took money from her wallet without asking, his excuse made sense. His friend had come to collect money for concert tickets, and she wasn't available. She felt annoyed*

nevertheless; his going into her wallet without asking violated her privacy.

Low self-esteem. Phrases like "I'm worthless," "I hate myself," and "I always mess up," become masks when they're used to hide and suppress anger toward oneself or someone else.

Passivity. A lack of assertiveness, a do-nothing attitude, can mask negative, passive-aggressive forms of anger. For example, "Let someone else do it," "I don't care to get involved," or "It won't make a difference, so why bother."

Road rage. This unique mask allows you to be mean and cruel, while remaining anonymous. No one will know it's you.

Other behaviors used to mask anger include extreme politeness, humor, laughter, sarcasm, criticism, judgments of self and others, illness, and fatigue. The anger underlying these masks has no place to go, so it remains in your body, creating muscular tension. The following exercise helps you bring your anger masks into conscious awareness, release them, and release the anger that underlies the masks. Before you do the exercise, list the ways you try to conceal your anger in your anger journal.

EXERCISE: Releasing Anger Masks

The exercise for releasing anger masks is the same as the one for Releasing Negative Thoughts, only the first bullet point differs.

- Name an anger mask you're ready to release, say it aloud, and write it in your journal. It could be blame, explanation, low self-esteem, or humor. Example: "I fell asleep and that's why dinner is late." (The explanation mask conceals her passive-aggressive behavior.)

The next four steps are the same as in the "Releasing Negative Thoughts" exercise. Refer to that exercise, described above. Do the exercise once a day for two weeks and then two or three times a week to let go of your anger masks. When you release the mask, you're releasing the underlying anger.

Next, information about blocked, toxic energy and why you need to release it from your body will be explored.

Letting Go of Stuck Energy

Your body's energy, like the gasoline in your car, keeps you going. It's meant to keep you vital and alive. It helps you live fully, love completely, be creative, think logically, and connect with others. It flows naturally along defined pathways called meridians and when it's used up, it releases through the aura, described in Eastern philosophy as an electromagnetic energy field surrounding and emanating from the body (Brennan 1988).

Although it's a neutral force, your energy is affected by your thinking and emotions. Positivity, such as joy, causes vibrant, alive, and fluid energy, whereas negativity, self-judgments, and criticism of others causes slower, stuck, constricted, and dense energy. Most of us have a combination of light and dark energy in our bodies. Kerri experienced both kinds of energy, one right after the other.

> When she entered the pool area, knowing that she had a good chance of winning the diving competition, Kerri danced onto the board, alive with pleasure. But when she couldn't get her husband's attention to film the event, she suddenly felt unimportant, and her energy collapsed. Even though she won the contest, she left the pool feeling deflated, conscious of how different her body felt after experiencing disappointment.

Think of energy as a continuum. At one end your energy flows easily and your body is relaxed, and at the other, it is slowed by muscles tight with blocked energy. When energy flows well, you can focus on achieving your goals. You can have that aha moment that leads to securing a new career, finishing a play, or conceiving a child. When your energy is blocked and out of balance, you experience toxic anger, frustrations, and the feeling of being stuck. You may feel overwhelmed, anxious, detached, bored, or empty. Heavy or stuck energy can lead to chaotic, unsatisfying relationships, bitter fights, or a desire to pull away and create distance.

Most of us fall somewhere in the middle on the energy continuum, between the extremes of being completely in balance and relaxed and being completely out of balance and blocked. We have a mix of both light and dark energy in our bodies. Some body parts reflect harmony and move gracefully, and others disharmony, unresolved anger, and move awkwardly. Correspondingly, some aspects of ourselves are creative and loving, whereas others view life as a struggle.

Engaging in exercises to release negative energy is an important part of self-care and managing burnout for women. Since negative thoughts and anger cause your energy to get stuck, try the following exercise to release energy held in contracted muscles throughout your body.

Staccato Breathing

This technique releases tension from your muscles, including the chest, arms, back, diaphragm, abdomen, pelvis, and legs. Because neurotransmitters release into your body during sleep, you awake with toxins in your body that may upset your equilibrium and cause anger. Beginning the day with this exercise helps you release and manage your anger throughout the day. During the exercise, your body expands and contracts, mimicking the biological pulsations of all living creatures (Pierrakos 1987, Wilner 1999).

Use this technique ten minutes a day, preferably in the morning, but it is helpful at any time. There are three stages to the breathing: inhaling, exhaling, and pausing (or relaxing). Pay attention to your physical sensations as you breathe.

- Lie on a couch, mat, or carpet with your feet flat, knees bent, and eyes closed.

- Inhale in short sniffs with your mouth closed to the count of five: One. Two. Three. Four. Five. At the same time...

- Arch your back (as you inhale through the nose), sticking your chest out and pressing your shoulders and pelvis into the floor. You should look like an inverted U. This step creates space between your back and the floor.

- Hold your breath for three seconds, then exhale through the mouth, vocalizing an "uuuhhh" sound.

- As you exhale, round your shoulders in toward your heart and tip the lower part of your pelvis up, an inch off the floor, taking the U shape. Feel your back flatten onto the floor. Your head can rest on the floor or lift up slightly as your shoulders roll forward.

- Relax for a few seconds and then begin the next breath.

Continue this fashion of breathing for ten minutes. When you stop, get up slowly and do one or two of the grounding exercises from Step Three.

Releasing Trauma and Abuse

When you've experienced trauma and abuse, your release of anger differs slightly from the exercises above. Because you need to reclaim parts of yourself that were taken from you while you were in a state of extreme fear, it's best to verbally release first by telling and retelling your story. This can occur in counseling or psychotherapy, with friends and family, or by yourself using a tape recorder. As difficult as it may be to share this experience, the more details you supply, including smells, sounds, colors, and actions, the faster you'll heal.

Next, because your body froze and detached from the situation, you need to free up your energy slowly and softly to release the underlying fear without retraumatizing yourself. This includes making tiny, gentle body movements, stretching, and self-massage. Your body may tremble or shake, positive signs that it's letting go. After you release fear, which may take several weeks, you may be ready to release anger. Stand up, imagine your perpetrator, stamp your feet, and say strongly, "I'm here, I exist." When you feel like fighting back, punch out in front of you or punch some pillows. You may scream. If you don't have privacy, scream or yell in the shower or in your car so that your screams won't affect other people. Remember to do grounding exercises before and after the anger release.

Ridding Yourself of What Keeps You Stuck

Healing from toxic anger involves letting go of negativity, breaking through blockages, and freeing energy so that it can flow throughout your body. By ridding yourself of the thoughts that create it, the masks you use to hide it, and the heavy energy that weighs you down, you empower yourself through assertive, honest, and direct communication, creating meaningful relationships and better health. As you attain a more relaxed and balanced lifestyle, and more pleasure, your need to rely on anger for strength diminishes. The next step, *Transform*, raises the vibration of the energy that has been released and converts your anger into a compassionate and loving force.

Transform: From Hotheaded to Warmhearted

Nothing changes in your life until the body's more integrated and it vibrates.

—John C. Pierrakos, *Core Energetics*

Georgette was an angel. She cared for anyone who touched her life. There was always a warm bed if they needed a place to stay and concert tickets to hear their favorite groups. She never forgot birthdays. Yet, when some small grudge grew into a monstrous problem, she stopped talking to her best friend for more than five years. Finally, she decided she didn't want to live with this hate any longer. She tacked a picture of her ex-friend on a wall, piled three strong pillows on a table in front of the picture, grabbed a plastic, dime-store bat, and wacked the pillows. As she hit, she looked at the picture, and angry words spilled out of her mouth. When she was spent, she cried; her body trembled and vibrated all over. This went on for an hour and then something changed inside of her. She looked at the picture and said, "I love you, I am so sorry. I forgive you." The next day, she called her friend and told her, "I don't want to live without you in my life." They made plans to get together the following week. It felt like a miracle.

By raising your energy's vibration, as Georgette did in the preceding example, you can transform your anger to love and compassion, freeing yourself from the grasp of negative, fear-based, angry thinking. Rhythmic movements, sound, dance, and work with the chakras are powerful methods used to transcend negative energy and change your energy from heavy to light.

Using Energy to Move from Anger to Love

Even if you can't see energy, all material things and beings, including you, are made up of it (Chopra and Kafatos 2018; Pierrakos 1987). It flows naturally through the muscles of your body, just like blood flows through your veins.

However, when you're angry or physiologically aroused, it changes its route through your body in response to what is stressing you, and it gets stuck in tense and bulging muscles. It remains locked in these muscles until you identify the emotions that are suppressed and release them. Then your energy flows again, your nervous system calms, and your anger transforms.

You can imagine the transformation process as four circles. In the outermost circle your energy is heavy and dark. Here lives toxic anger, denial, suppression, and the desire to act out destructively. Inside that circle is another circle, or layer, that represents the original wound. This hurt goes back to your childhood. As you do the assigned exercises and move your body, you release suppressed emotions and clogged energy. In the third circle, while continuing to move, you own your anger and take responsibility for it. This circle represents your constructive anger. Finally, when your energy vibrates at a higher frequency, you experience true compassion and love, the innermost and fourth circle.

As you move from circle to circle, or layer to layer, your emotions change; what once had the power to destroy enhances your life. In the innermost circle, you experience several forms of love, including romantic, platonic, spiritual, transpersonal, filial, and familiar. Here's a description of Juanita's transformation process.

Juanita's suppressed anger toward her ex-husband verged on hate. Because she couldn't communicate with him without fighting, she sought sole custody of their three children, aged seven through twelve. But he fought back and was granted custody because the children told the court that they preferred to live with their dad. This was a wake-up call for Juanita. She recognized that she needed to do something about her anger to regain her children's love. Body awareness, owning her anger, and energy and chakra work helped her open and unlock her closed heart. By the time they were teens, the children wanted to spend as much time with Juanita, who had remarried, as with their father.

An exercise using three pillows demonstrates how this transformation process works (Pierrakos 1987).

EXERCISE: Three Pillows—Blame, Anger, Truth

Think of someone who recently triggered your anger. Do the exercise with this person in mind.

- Place three chairs in a row and put a different colored pillow on each. Label the pillows: Blame, Anger, and Truth.

- Begin by sitting on the Blame chair. Imagine the person you're angry with sitting across from you. Tell this person each injustice you experienced at this person's hands.

- Now move to the Anger chair. Envision the same person. Direct your darkest anger toward them, saying either, "I am angry with you," "I hate you," "I resent you," "I want to hurt you," "I want to destroy you," or "I want to see you suffer." You can also make growling sounds if the words do not come.

- When your anger feels genuine and free of blame, move to pillow number three, the Truth chair. No longer guided by anger, blame, or negative thoughts, your heart can thaw, and you can experience gratitude, peace, or pleasure. Face the person and with a soft heart, describe one or more positive feelings you have toward him or her. If your heart doesn't soften, don't force it: go back to the Blame and Anger pillows and repeat the exercise until your heart prepares to open.

Next, I would like you to consider another way to transform toxic anger to love: by adding more pleasure to your life and balancing your energy.

Pleasure Helps Transform Anger to Love

Let's look at the role pleasure plays in transforming anger. Pleasure is associated with positive emotions and activities that stimulate the brain's reward center. When you experience pleasure, the neurotransmitter dopamine is released into the brain, you feel good, and you're more likely to be compassionate and giving to others. Feeling pleasure motivates you to forgive others and let go of old, painful, and anger-producing stories.

However, through the ages women have been taught that too much pleasure is bad. If you go out dancing, you may come home pregnant; if you're happy when pregnant, you may have a miscarriage; if you are joyful and do things for pleasure, you are selfish or even worse, a narcissist. Some religious groups connect worldly pleasures to sin and most people, including children, learn that loss feels more painful when it follows joy and love. The fear of pleasure is so enculturated that you may have grown up believing that it is better to be somewhat unhappy, neutral, or angry than joyful and happy.

However, the opposite is true; pleasure, leisure time activities, and quality of life are associated with lower blood pressure and lower arousal (Rein, Atkinson, and McCraty 1995). Pleasure, contentment, and joy occur when you relax and your body moves freely and naturally. Behavioral scientists teach that pleasure and anger aren't experienced simultaneously; if you're angry, you can't feel pleasure, and if you're in good spirits, anger has trouble getting in the door. Here are some additional facts:

- Toxic anger sometimes feels good, but you're experiencing negative excitement, not pleasure.

- Feeling pleasure is necessary for self-realization, healing, and personal growth to occur.

- You can't experience pleasure if you're cut off from your body.

- Pleasure is associated with a more meaningful and fulfilling life.

- Rational anger, shared appropriately, provides pleasure.

- If your life is out of balance, you won't experience pleasure.

Balance is important for experiencing pleasure and transforming toxic anger. The next section explores why.

The Problem with Being Out-of-Balance

Ancient Chinese philosophers say that your assertive yang energy and receptive yin energy must be balanced to achieve health and happiness. Yang, a powerful energy, makes things happen, initiates activities, and takes the lead. Yin, a receptive energy, comes into play when you soften and relax; you accept an invitation, knit a scarf, or hug your children. Toxic anger creates an imbalance. The assertive yang energy becomes aggressive, controlling, and demanding of others and if you suppress your anger, even your receptive, yin energy turns against you, leading to health issues, passive-aggressive behavior, and unhappiness.

When it comes to anger, women have often been out of balance. In the distant past, they had too much passive yin energy. Men led and women followed, perhaps secretly resenting it. Now, the balance has swung in the other direction. Much like men, women today are overly active. The current superwomen have too little time to relax or focus on self-care. Most likely, you push yourself hard working a job, running a household, and planning social events. Overreliance on yang energy leads to stress, bouts of anger, and burnout. In this example, Sarah has too much yang energy:

A divorced mother of two, ages seven and ten, Sarah regularly screamed at her children in the evening, Afterward, she would feel intense guilt and apologize. She worked full time as a legal secretary. In addition to her regular assignments, her boss relied on her to respond to phone calls, make airplane reservations, and order takeout. It was her responsibility to get the children to and from school and to their extracurricular activities. She pushed forward, crossing each thing off her list, shutting down her emotions so she could get things done. By eight at night, she would fall apart and become her worst self.

If, on the other hand, you suppress anger, you have too much negative yin or passive energy. Here's what happened to Beth:

Beth, a clinical social worker, spent eight hours a day with clients and worked on weekends too. She enjoyed helping people, but born poor, she felt she had to work. Her suppressed anger sprang from the belief that she had gotten the short end of the stick. When rheumatoid arthritis hit, the pain was so debilitating that she was forced to pay attention to her needs and seek help for her anger.

Both Sarah and Beth, like many of us, need more balance in their lives. This imbalance shows up in your nervous system as well. The sympathetic nervous system is behind the tension you experience when you push hard to succeed at a project or suppress anger in tight muscles. Its partner, the parasympathetic nervous system, does the opposite; its message is about relaxation, letting go, lying in the sun, muscles releasing. Imagine how different Sarah's and Beth's lives would be, and ours too, if their sympathetic and parasympathetic nervous systems were balanced and they added pleasurable activities into their daily routine.

Transforming your toxic anger, adding pleasure, and attaining balance can be achieved through movement.

Rhythmic Movement

Rhythmic movement is found throughout nature, in the migratory route of birds, menstrual cycles, and heartbeats. Shamans use rhythmic drumming to enter alternative states of consciousness and initiate healing practices. It can transform anger and bring pleasure into your life. It creates pulsations that sustain healing states in your body. You can tap into waves of pulsating sound to change hateful feelings. That's what happened to Jeannette:

> Jeannette had a vague memory of her father reading her fairytales. But mostly she remembered him rejecting her after losing his job and falling into a deep depression. She blamed and resented him for this. At a drumming circle, she picked up a drum and beat it, moving along with the fast rhythm, Then, she saw him in a new light. She envisioned this depressed man turning to her mother for support. She saw them hug and hold each other. Now, she could let go of her anger and say goodbye with love. She was ready to build healthy relationships of her own.

Sluggish energy, resulting from negative thinking, fear, and anger, transforms when sound and movement increase in speed and intensity. Your energy vibrates at a higher frequency, an important ingredient in the transformation process. Dance, like drumming, has this effect. Here's what Lucia experienced:

> Lucia, who waitressed at the local diner, did well in tips. To keep her customers happy, she smiled and had a jolly word for everyone, even those whose behavior was demeaning or sexually inappropriate. On the inside, she seethed toward some of these "low lives." When she attended a country and western dance with her husband, everything changed. As she stamped her feet to the music, she envisioned stamping on the heads of customers who treated her poorly. As she let her anger go, it was replaced by pleasure, the joy of movement, and feeling one with the music. At the end of the evening, free of negativity and refreshed, she decided to sign up for country and western dance classes. After several weeks, she was able to tell inappropriate customers that unless their behavior changed, they would have to dine elsewhere.

The following exercise will help you explore and transform your anger through dance.

EXERCISE: Dancing Your Anger

Think of someone or something that triggered your anger recently. Design a dance to portray the situation, responding to whatever occurred with powerful and forceful movements. Move to rhythmic music, pop, hip-hop, heart beats, American Indian or shamanic drumming, country and western, Latin, or reggae. Write about the experience of "dancing your anger" in your journal and note whether your feelings changed as you danced.

Strong Movement

Strong movement helps your anger transform as well. Unblocking energy locked in your muscles, releasing suppressed emotion and raising its vibration, can bring about a major turnaround.

EXERCISE: Strong Movement with Towel or Scarf

Think of an anger experience from the past or present. Remember the specific details, your feelings, and the person who triggered you.

- Start by grounding. Standing with your feet shoulder width apart, bend your knees into a half-squat, and return to a straight-legged position by pushing your feet hard against the floor. Do this fast, until your legs begin to tremble, a sign that your energy is flowing.

- Now, roll up a towel or a scarf and begin to twist it with both hands as if you are strangling someone or something. This may feel strange, but it works. As you twist, make sounds or express whatever comes up for you. You may experience emotions such as anger, sadness, fear, or shame. Welcome them without judgment.

- When you stop, envision the person who triggered your anger in your mind's eye. Think of several positive qualities to describe this person and say or think them as you reach out with open arms.

This exercise raises your energy's vibratory frequency, and at the same time transforms the heavy energy associated with dark anger to compassion and love.

Chakra Movement

Moving your chakra energy is another way to transform toxic anger. Fresh energy from the universe enters your body through twelve energy centers called chakras (Brennan 1988; Pierrakos 1987).

Their energy nourishes your whole being and then releases through your aura, the subtle energy that surrounds your body. Each chakra plays a role in raising your body's natural vibrations. Following is a description of the chakras. Refer back to the "Placement & Meaning of the Chakras" diagram on page 86 if you would like a visual guide.

The highest center, the cosmic center, resides at the top of your head toward the front. The first center, the root chakra, sits toward the rear of the pelvic floor. Five pairs are located in between, one in the front and the other in the back of your body. Those in the back represent taking action, whereas those in the front are associated with feelings. When your energy flows well, each chakra plays a role.

The root chakra represents safety and security. Its color is red, and it's connected to the feet, hands, and glands that produce estrogen and testosterone. It helps you ground your anger and bring the heat of arousal away from your head and chest, down toward your legs and feet.

The pair of chakras, 2a and 2b, are associated with pleasure, vitality, and sexuality. Chakra 2a sits on the front between your hips and helps you feel pleasure. Chakra 2b, on your lower back, reflects your willingness to engage in pleasurable activities. They both radiate orange energy and connect to your ankles, wrists, and adrenal glands—the glands that manage stress in your body, regulate your immune system, and control your blood pressure.

Chakra 3a is the self-center. It's a large, bright yellow chakra located in the middle of your solar plexus, and it connects to your calves, forearms, and buttocks. It flows well when your life path and goals are free of negative energy. It pairs with 3b, the healing center, located on your lower back above the sacrum. Known for its purple-colored energy, this center flourishes and radiates good health as you let go of toxic anger.

Chakras 4a and 4b have to do with love and power. In the center of your chest, the heart chakra, 4a, releases pastel pink and green energy and connects to your elbows, knees, thymus gland, and immune system. Energy flow at this chakra enhances your ability to feel love and compassion. When you're hurt, frightened, or angry, you build protective walls around your heart, diminishing its energy flow.

The heart chakra's partner, 4b, flows well when you feel assertive and empowered. It is located on the back between the shoulder blades, and the color of its energy is bright red. When angry, it contracts and becomes overly controlling and demanding or the opposite, passive, collapsed, and ready to give up. When your energy is balanced, it works with the heart, integrating power and compassion. I call this the "active heart."

Bright blue chakra 5a represents your voice and throat center. Located midpoint on the throat, it connects to the thyroid gland. Flowing well, you communicate your true feelings, speak assertively, and receive, listen, or take in feedback. Aggressive or suppressed anger causes your throat muscles to contract, whereas speaking reasonably and listening to another's point of view relaxes these muscles. Chakra 5b, its partner located at the nape of the neck, is called the executive center and has yellow energy. Flowing well, it keeps you organized and helps with administrative tasks, allowing you to feel in control and less chaotic, overwhelmed, or impatient.

Chakra 6a represents your third eye or intuition, and 6b your old brain. In the middle of your forehead, 6a, an indigo color, connects to the pituitary gland. When it flows well, it facilitates your sixth sense, intuition, and awareness. Listening to it helps you follow the right path and know when you're safe and free of danger. Its partner, 6b, radiating yellow energy, is positioned in the middle of the back of the head and connects to the hypothalamus, which controls automatic functions in the body—this includes eating and sleeping—as well as to the limbic system, the home of the fight and flight response. Energy flowing well here can free you from experiencing unnecessary arousal. Simply pat the back of the head on occasion to clear this center.

The energy of the 7th chakra, the crown chakra at the top of your head, is white. When the energy flows well, it represents the pineal gland and spirituality. Meditation, positive thoughts, prayer, and forgiveness are tools associated with this chakra that help you remain calm and transform your toxic anger.

Do the following chakra exercise to move your energy, raise its vibration, and transform you anger to love, compassion, and gratitude.

EXERCISE: Spinning Chakras

Do this exercise every day for two weeks, then twice a week for two more weeks.

1. Stand or sit, quieting your mind and grounding, feet shoulder width apart, facing forward, and knees slightly bent. At first, you may want to do this exercise in front of a mirror to locate the position of each chakra.

2. Move your hand to your root chakra. Imagine the bright red color. Quickly make small clockwise circles with your hand in front of this energy center. (If making circles is difficult, wave your hand back and forth in front of the chakra.) Do this for a minute, then shut your eyes, breathe slowly, and stay centered. Think of feeling safe and secure.

3. Bring your hand to 6a, the pelvic chakra. Imagine the bright orange color. Make small clockwise circles, moving your hand quickly in front of this center. Do this for a minute. Then shut your eyes, breathe slowly, and stay centered. Think of your ability to experience pleasure and vitality.

4. Proceed to 5a, the solar plexus. Imagine its bright yellow color. Make small, fast clockwise circles with your hand in front of this center. Do

this for a minute and then shut your eyes, breathe slowly, and stay centered. Think of your life path and what you would like to accomplish in the future.

5. Focus on the heart chakra, 4a. Imagine pastel pink and green colors emanating from your chest. Make small clockwise circles with your hand moving quickly in front of this center. Do this for a minute and then shut your eyes, breathe slowly, and stay centered. Connect to your heart and think of love, compassion, and positive feelings.

6. Bring you hand to your throat, 3a, and imagine the vibrant blue color of its energy. Make small, clockwise circles, moving your hand quickly in front of this energy center. Do this for a minute, then shut your eyes, breath slowly, and stay centered. Think of speaking about your anger rationally and being in your truth.

7. Advance your hand to 2a, the third eye. The color is indigo. Make small, fast, clockwise circles with your hand in front of this energy center. Do this for a minute, then shut your eyes, breathe slowly, and stay centered. Think of your intuition and sixth sense leading you toward peace, pleasure, and fulfillment.

8. End with the crown chakra, at the top of your head, visualizing its white energy. Making small clockwise circles with your hand, move it quickly above this energy center. Do this for a minute, then shut your eyes, breathe slowly, and stay centered. Think of being in truth, entertaining forgiveness, and feeling compassion.

Do this chakra exercise to clear and transform your energy or whenever you want to feel fabulous.

The last exercise is a meditation that focuses on transforming your anger as you watch it float away.

EXERCISE: Anger Transformation Meditation

Sitting quietly, focus on your breathing and imagine yourself in a beautiful spot near a pond filled with clear water. The sun shines on you, the breeze touches your skin gently, and butterflies flit from flower to flower. Having brought your anger here to purify it, envision letting go of your destructive urges and bitter, hostile thoughts. Drop them into the clear water and watch them float away. Feel lighter as you free yourself of this negativity. If you have been an aggressive, Anger-Out person, your dragon breath is gone. And if you withheld your anger so that your unspoken thoughts poisoned the atmosphere, imagine yourself ready to express them. Experience a deep sense of peace in this beautiful spot. Recognize your anger as part of nature, like the butterflies, to be accepted, understood, and transformed. Entertain compassion for your adversaries and send them heartfelt energy.

From Toxic Anger to Pleasure and Love

Through movement, you can change the frequency at which your energy vibrates, and in doing so, let go of toxic anger and replace it with pleasure, compassion, acceptance, and understanding. Rhythmic movements, sound, dance, and spinning the chakras are powerful methods used to overcome the consequences of negative energy and change your energy from dark to light. In the next step, you will explore methods to communicate anger in reasonable and appropriate ways and build connections between people.

STEP SIX

Share to Spare: Build Bridges to Repair

As people reveal themselves, they heal themselves.

—Caroline Myss

After an Al-Anon meeting, Heidi, age forty-three, decided to confront her mother. She needed to tell her she was angry, but she didn't know how. There was so much yelling in her house growing up, she held everything in as an adult, not wanting to be like them. But it was time. While driving to her mother's apartment, she wondered what she would say. Though she feared the response she would get, she entered the apartment and said, "I need to speak to you about my anger." It wasn't as hard as she thought. Her mother, now fifteen years sober and having done some therapy, responded, "I've been expecting this conversation."

Heidi said, "I'm angry with you because I never knew which mother to expect. You could be the cuddly woman who held me close when I had a fever or a scary witch with flashing eyes and fangs. I'm angry with you for pushing my sister down the stairs and making me watch. I'm angry at you for forcing me to sleep under the bed without blankets. I'm angry with you for throwing a plate at me. I am so angry at you." Her mother listened and when she finished, said, "I'm so sorry. If I could change any of those things, I would. I hope that you can accept my apology."

It's difficult for women to share negative feelings. Sometimes you're over-whelmed with emotion and you don't know where to start. At other times, you stop yourself from sharing your anger because you don't know what to say and you don't have the vocabulary to discuss it rationally. You're concerned about hurting the other person, so you hope the situation will go away and be forgotten or overlooked. If you do say some-thing, you wonder if the relationship will ever recover, or if you will lose this friend, daughter, son, husband, colleague, or relative, forever. You also don't want to be seen as someone who is out of control or volatile. You haven't had the life experiences to teach you that sharing your anger will bring you authenticity, better health, and closer relationships.

Yet anger, when not toxic, is healthy. It motivates you to express your ideas and opinions and share what is truly important to you. However, because it's an emotion, it differs across individuals depending on their biological makeup and past experiences. Whereas you may yell and slam doors when aroused, your best friend, under the same circum-stances, may appear calm. Or you consider an insult the worst thing that could happen to you and your spouse says, "Why are you letting that little thing bother you?"

Anger Equals Differences of Opinion

Picture an elephant: its long, curving trunk; tusks; large, flappy ears; gray, mottled skin; thick legs; big feet; full, powerful body; and spindly tail. One part may grab your interest and some other part might fasci-nate another person. Anger is like that. You are both looking at differ-ent facets of a situation. Since you may each be right about the part you're looking at, it's important to have a discussion and to hear the other's point of view.

However, even when you're reasonable and trying to reach a com-promise, the opposition may be unwilling to give an inch. Healthy com-munication about anger means you're able to tolerate someone else's bad behavior and not match it. On occasion, no matter how hard you try, the other may not be open to discussion or negotiation. There is no need to capitulate, but you don't have to react with rage either. You can agree to disagree.

When you share your anger with the person with whom you're angry, the goal is to be authentic and bring reasonable, rational, open, and honest content to the conversation. When you use your frontal lobes, the part of the brain that houses logic, you are more likely to reach a resolution. To set this discussion up for success, schedule it for a time and place that works for both of you. Leave your expectations for how it should go behind, stay present, and be aware of your body as well as your mind. Be prepared to listen as well as state your case. Realize that most people feel criticized when you bring a problem to their attention, so don't expect a positive response to what you have to say. Say it, hear the response, think about the other's point of view, and respond with reasonable alternatives or a simple "I'm sorry" or "let me think about it."

Why Communicating About Anger Fails

A bridge symbolizes joining two or more objects together; it is designed to connect two points. However, bridges break: just as in the nursery rhyme "London Bridge Is Falling Down." Some versions of its lyrics suggest that a bridge breaks when "sticks and stones" can't hold it up, when "wood and clay...melt away," and when "iron and steel...bend and break." With toxic anger, your relationships, like London Bridge, are at risk of breaking or being torn asunder. It helps to consider whether your anger, even when hidden, may have jeopardized past relationships with ex-partners, friends, or colleagues who experienced you as negative, were scared by your anger, or were hurt too much.

Additionally, you may have jeopardized your relationship with yourself. If you denied your anger to maintain peace or appear neutral, you betrayed yourself by not standing up for your beliefs. Although this may seem minor, denying your anger over and over could lead to feeling weak and self-disgust.

When you say something hurtful or turn your back on someone, you loosen positive bonds. Dark anger uses blame, criticism, and judgments to communicate. It employs tone of voice to make others feel bad. Even if the words are pleasant, your jaw tightens and your voice gets quiet or shrill. Sneers, slit eyes, tight lips, and confrontational body movements such as "getting in someone's face," which occurs when you cross into another's physical space, all have negative consequences for relationships.

Joan, who is on the verge of another breakup, describes herself as an expert at negative nonverbals, saying,

> I grew up in a home where "talking back," or even having a different opinion, to a hostile, angry parent was not an option. I learned two behaviors that hurt my relationships later in life. The first was twisting my lips in such a way as to say, "You have no idea what you're talking about," and the second was rolling my eyes when I disagreed.

Sneers and eyerolls, nonverbal expressions that show contempt, can end relationships. Statistics show that when partners feel demeaned or disrespected, illnesses occur and relationships have less chance of surviving (Gottman and Levenson 2000; Malarkey et al. 1994).

Other research indicates that humans don't have an accurate view of how they're perceived by others (Burns 1999). Along these lines, you may not realize how others perceive you when you're angry or how they receive your anger. If you suppress anger, you may think they don't notice, but they do.

Here are some common toxic communication patterns:

My Way or the Highway—Willful, Aggressive, and Needing to Be Right

If you need to be right because you trust your own thinking over that of other people or it helps you feel better about yourself, you may get angry when people don't agree with you. Your need makes you competitive, focused on winning, and less able to resolve problems and build bridges. Edwina could not get past this need.

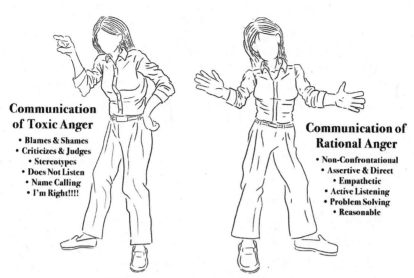

Communication of Toxic Anger
- Blames & Shames
- Criticizes & Judges
- Stereotypes
- Does Not Listen
- Name Calling
- I'm Right!!!!

Communication of Rational Anger
- Non-Confrontational
- Assertive & Direct
- Empathetic
- Active Listening
- Problem Solving
- Reasonable

Differences in Communication Styles

Edwina, a tall, broad-shouldered woman with flashing eyes and a ponytail, loomed over her adult daughter. She expected Petra to agree to prepare a holiday dinner for twelve. When Petra, tired from a semester of teaching, didn't agree to take this on, Edwina's eyes narrowed and she began to cut Petra off. Then she grew cold and distant, never asking for Petra's point of view.

You may know women like Edwina who can't compromise or take no for an answer. By letting go of your need to be right, you have an opportunity to see the world though someone else's eyes and be more compassionate.

Blame and Judgment

Although judgment and criticism can be constructive, sometimes they're not given or received that way. If you point out mistakes with hostility, which is what happens with blame, it defeats your purpose—which is to resolve a problem—and it triggers hurt and anger in the other. Try making a request instead. Here's how they differ:

Snarling: "You didn't close the refrigerator door again."

Requesting: "Can you get that door, please?"

Blame occurs when you hold someone else responsible for a situation without taking responsibility for your part; you make your anger and your upset the other's fault. Janet and Phil played the blame game:

Janet blamed Phil for staying late at work and not paying attention to her when he got home. He counterattacked, referring to a stack of unpaid bills, and criticized her for overspending. Each substituted blame for anger, never having to say "I feel angry with you." Their blaming behavior took the place of an open and honest discussion about their differences, leading each to secretly think of divorce. When they learned to share their anger and listen to the other's point of view, they were more loving and one hundredfold happier.

It's important to share feelings about situations that trigger your anger without making it the other's fault. If you find yourself blaming or criticizing another, recognize your negativity and do something about it. A thought stopping exercise like snapping a rubber band on your wrist each time you start to say something critical works well. Or let out a deep, slow breath, as if you're blowing through a straw, before offering your critique, which gives you time to reframe your comments and say something more positive. Here's an example:

Criticism (voice rising): "How come you're not in graduate school?"

Support: "I think you'll make the right choice. Sometimes it takes time to know the next step."

Humiliating and Shaming—There's Something Wrong with You

When you humiliate or shame someone with your anger, you intend to degrade or embarrass the person. If you are in a rage or acting out passive-aggressively, your desire to get back may take this form. Attacking someone's character derives from jealousy, envy, and a need to exert power. Bernice realized that she had acted this way at a recent book group meeting.

After Lily shared a memory triggered by the book they were reading, Bernice told her that she sounded like a victim and that she should have stood up and fought. Feeling embarrassed, Lily wrote a letter withdrawing from the book group. When Bernice realized her comments were a factor in Lily's departure, she called Lily and apologized. Later she recognized that her criticism had more to do with her own life than Lily's.

Changing Another Person

You can't use anger to change someone, even when you wish that person were different. When people change, it's because they are willing and motivated to be different. Accept the people in your life as they are; if they're toxic, end the relationship and move on. If there're reasons you can't terminate the relationship, detach yourself from the negative energy they exude, but forgive them so that your anger toward them doesn't turn against yourself.

An Eye for an Eye: You'll Get What You Deserve

If you subscribe to the "eye for an eye" brand of problem-solving and prefer to get back rather than have honest communications and forgive, you will continue to carry unresolved anger in your bodymind.

Mary shared that in a fit of anger, she threw a book at her mother while yelling, "Now you get what you deserve." Her mother's arm was black and blue for a month. When she saw what her rage could do, she joined an anger group, saying that was the last time she would throw something at another person.

Categorizing People: Using Stereotypes

Try not to use your anger to depersonalize people or treat them like objects. This can occur if you categorize people according to gender, religion, ethnicity, disability, race, religion, or socioeconomic class. Phrases like "those people," "people like that," and "that type of person" have a negative cast and ignore individual differences. Maria found herself guilty of this:

> When teaching a parenting class, she inferred that fathers are unable to nurture due to their lack of oxytocin, the love hormone, an essential hormone for childbirth and breastfeeding. She didn't account for the fact that men differ in their nurturing abilities.

Attacking Close Family Members or People in Your Intimate Circle

Try not to express toxic anger toward close family members. It creates dysfunctional relationships, tension, lack of support, and loneliness. If you're friendly and polite with strangers and acquaintances when you disagree but ready for an argument over small matters, as well as large ones, within the family circle, you're giving yourself permission to be your worst self in this environment. Because you live in close proximity and spend more time together, you are more likely to have disagreements. Your closest relationships may become contentious and unpleasant unless you provide opportunities to discuss these differences, listen to each other, forgive, and apologize.

Women who vent rage get angrier, not less angry, creating even more tension and more enemies. Yet when you withhold and suppress anger, you grow bitter, cranky, and embattled. You have less joy and can possibly develop health issues. The goal is to find a middle ground: to express yourself assertively without causing harm. By being honest, direct, and tactful when expressing anger, a resolution may be in sight. Do the following self-analysis to estimate the effect of toxic anger on your past relationships.

EXERCISE: Self-Analysis

In your journal, using the four-point scale (0 = No Effect; 1 = Minor Effect; 2 = Moderate Effect; 3 = Major Effect), rate the impact your anger has had on your relationships with the following people:

mother	father	parental figures
siblings	children	in-laws
relatives	spouse	partner
ex-partners	partner's children	pets
friends	romantic interests	medical professionals
shopkeepers	teachers	colleagues
bosses	employees	neighbors
customers	yourself	religious leaders
drivers	police	military
authority figures	customer service personnel	

The next section focuses on learning how to share and communicate your anger positively. You may find some of these ideas familiar and others totally new.

Communicating Anger Positively

Women wonder how they can communicate anger and still be seen in a positive light. Here are some pointers that will help you share your anger effectively:

Take full responsibility for your anger. Acknowledge that your anger comes from you and it's not the fault of the other person. Remind yourself it's due to your brain, upbringing, nervous system, and genetics. Someone else with a different brain and history will react differently in the same situation. When you take responsibility, others can hear your message without having to defend themselves, resulting in a greater understanding and an eventual meeting of the minds.

Be a great listener even when you don't agree. Engage in active listening: put your point of view and thoughts aside in order to repeat back with understanding what the other communicated. As you listen, focus on the speaker's main point, and then share your understanding of what was said, checking to make sure you heard it right. Sometimes, the reply will be, "Yes, that is exactly what I think," and at other times, you will hear, "No, that is not quite right, here's what I was trying to say…" By listening, you give those with opposing views an opportunity to express themselves.

Be nonconfrontational when expressing anger. Here is a way to express anger that creates less friction. The formula to express anger without creating more discord involves saying something like, "When you do X, I feel Y, because of Z." You're aware that the other is doing something that triggers you, but it's not that person's fault you're triggered. Your nervous system responds to what that person is doing. For example, when my partner turns on the television when I am working, I am triggered. It's not their fault I'm annoyed and that I feel disrespected—my feelings go back to hurtful events from my childhood. Rather than blame them, I can request that they turn down the volume or ask me for my preference before turning the television on. Using the above formula, I could say, "When you turned on the television without telling me, I felt invisible and hurt because you didn't check if that would be okay for me."

EXERCISE: Using the Nonconfrontational Formula

In your journal list three incidents that irritated or annoyed you this week. Imagine yourself responding to each using the sentence pattern "when you did x, I felt y, because of z." Write the sentences in your journal.

Be assertive. When you're assertive, you empower yourself. Expressing anger assertively means being direct, clear, and truthful. Make "I" statements, not "you" statements. Rather than being angry, state clearly what you need from the other person. For example, if you're annoyed with your partner for coming home late, rather than saying, "You are selfish and inconsiderate," which would start an argument, you can state assertively, "When you came home late, I felt upset because I couldn't prepare for my class. I do need you to be on time tomorrow so I can grade papers and make dinner." Assertive statements contain facts, feelings, and needs: what the other did (fact), what you felt (feeling), and what you need (behavior) (McKay, Rogers, and McKay 2003).

EXERCISE: Expressing Yourself Assertively

In your journal, describe a recent event that triggered your anger. Using the assertive communication formula (fact, feeling, need), write a sentence stating the facts, what you felt, and what you need the other to do the next time the situation occurs.

Be actively empathic. When you're ready to share your anger with the other, be empathetic. Being empathetic means you're aware of the other's perceptions, feelings, and experiences. Even if it's not natural to you, empathy can be developed. You can use your imagination and make up what the other person is most likely experiencing and feeling. You can also ask questions to elicit her point of view. Or you can say, (1) "I imagine you are feeling… (fill in what she's feeling)" (2) "because… (fill in why you think she's having that experience)." Here's an example: "It seems like you feel misunderstood because you think you have been wrongly accused."

EXERCISE: Expressing Empathy When Angry

In your journal, describe a recent incident that incited your anger. Then, starting with "I imagine you're feeling…" express in one sentence what you believe the other was feeling and experiencing.

Consider practicalities. Choose a time that is acceptable to all parties for a discussion. Set boundaries for a safe and fair discussion. Think about whether it should occur in public (café or restaurant) or private (home or office). An automobile is not a good option for this discussion, unless it's parked. Decide whether there should be a time limit and whether it would be helpful to have a mediator present. Be willing to take a break if the discussion is not going well or postpone it if necessary.

Build a strength sandwich. If you need to give negative feedback or critique someone's behavior, try making a strength sandwich: first you say something positive, then something negative, and end with something positive. Here's an example of a strength sandwich from supervisor to supervisee:

> *You listened well and Joe felt heard. However, your response went over his head; you sounded a bit like a textbook. What you did at the end was great. He left feeling hopeful.*

Utilize the fifty-fifty rule. You take fifty percent of the responsibility for the problem or situation. When looked at objectively, both of you share some responsibility for the problem. Ask yourself, "What fifty percent is my responsibility?" For instance:

> *When Sheila expressed annoyance with Sheyanna for running out of the room during a violent episode, interrupting the movie, Sheyanna took responsibility. She hadn't shared her difficulties with violence with Sheila prior to this incident.*

EXERCISE: Describing Your Fifty Percent

Using one of the anger incidents in your journal, describe your part in what occurred.

Be positive. Show appreciation for the opportunity to talk about what is bothering you. Example: "I am pleased that I have had the opportunity to speak to you about this and that you were willing to listen to my point of view." Or if you were both angry, "I appreciate being able to speak honestly with each other about our differences."

Minimize arousal. Generally, your brain functions well; it's the home of logical thinking, perception, and memory, but when you're upset and angry, your fight or flight response is in charge. It relegates logic to the passenger seat, and you need to wait for physiological arousal to decrease and logic to move into the driver's seat before you can discuss the situation rationally. For some, it is a matter of minutes, for others, hours, and yet for others, days. Often with couples or family members, your timing is different. You may be ready to talk while your partner is still huffing and puffing or locked in the bathroom. You must wait until that person is ready, even when you're eager to mend the relationship.

Display agreeableness. When you speak, pay attention to your vocabulary because every word has power. Try to speak in a style similar to your opponent's so as to increase connectedness and achieve a more favorable outcome. Anger sometimes causes people to use a style or vocabulary that is not their norm, such as slang or four-letter words. Don't fall into this rut. At the same time, don't use the *exact* same vocabulary because she may think that you're making fun of her.

Receiving others' anger. When you share your anger, the recipient will likely respond defensively. Try not to reply with more anger, as that would be like pouring oil on flames. Instead, take a neutral stance. You might say, "I understand how you feel that way."

Put safety first. Know when to cancel, delay, or postpone a discussion concerning anger. Use nonverbal cues to predict the level of arousal in order to decide whether to proceed or wait until another time. If there is no eye contact, or if the person is leaning away from you, it may not be safe to talk. Very tight muscles mean the person could explode in rage. Look for tight jaws, fists, and tension throughout the body—a rubber band ready to snap. In that case, give the other space and distance. Recognize lack of conciliatory behavior by the choice of words and the loudness of the voice; screaming or whispering may indicate unresolved rage. By knowing what anger looks like in others, as well as in yourself, you can perceive when the time is right for communication.

Sharing anger electronically. The world has changed in terms of communications. You may use email and text more often to share your thoughts and feelings. When it comes to communicating anger, face-to-face communication may be the best alternative because texts and emails leave out nonverbal cues. You don't have the benefit of facial expression, body movement, or gesture to know how the conversation is progressing. And communications researchers say that nonverbal is 60 percent of the message (Birdwhistell 1970). Therefore, it's easier to be misunderstood. If you can't be in the same room, video platforms like Zoom, FaceTime, or WhatsApp are preferred.

However, some of these conversations will most likely occur electronically. If you do decide that text or email is your only choice, my advice is to have someone, your close friend or partner, read it and edit it before you hit send. Because if you regret what you wrote in the heat of emotion, it will be too late to change course. Electronic communication can also seem impersonal, so that empathy and compassion, so necessary when you deal with disagreements, don't come across.

Nevertheless, texts or email can work well if you don't act impulsively and aren't under the influence of toxic anger. You can choose your words carefully to avoid misunderstandings and you have more time to reflect on what you want to say. Since you can't see the other person, you don't have to react to her reactions to you. Also, you have a record of what was said, which can help if there is disagreement about the content.

The use of emojis. These are small digital images used to express emotions electronically. They may create problems if what you had in mind is understood differently by the receiver. Be cautious in using them. Those used to express disagreement include an angry or pouting face, a face with steam coming out of the nose, and a face with horns coming out of the head. They work if you're on the same page, and understand what the sender means, but can make things worse if you're not.

Don't overdo it. Even if you do everything right when it comes to communicating anger, if you share it every time you disagree, it may be a smidge too much. You could be seen as an "angry woman." However, this is not likely to happen if you continue to work on decreasing your negative thinking. Finding balance is important; letting a few things slide while sharing what matters most is absolutely necessary.

Using Anger to Build Bridges

Not only can your anger lead to positive communication experiences and creative problem solving, but it can also bring you closer to the person who triggered you. When you no longer need to be right, and you free your vocabulary from blame, judgment, and criticism, it offers the possibility of working together. It provides you with an opportunity to express your views honestly, even if the other person does not agree, and to hear another's position. By improving the manner you discuss anger, and waiting until it's safe to share, you open the doors to more pleasure and greater health. Your nervous system is more relaxed and the level of physiological arousal reduces in your body. You are now ready to move on to the final step of this seven-step anger transformation process, radical forgiveness.

Transcend: Experiencing Radical Forgiveness

We need to accept our human condition and then bit-by-bit discover that we are more than human.

—Donavan Thesenga, *Fear No Evil*

"I forgive you" is one of the most powerful statements you will ever make. In this step you will learn to forgive yourself and others by using somatic exercises including opening the heart, meditation, mindfulness, breathwork, and prayer, which are all supported by empirical research. They will help you cleanse your body of the negative chemistry left from toxic anger. Forgiveness assists you in letting go of the past and beginning a new chapter.

When you can't forgive, even with good reason, you continue to create negativity, and your body retains noxious chemicals that would have normally been released in minutes. You also carry with you heavy emotions associated with victimization, helplessness, and a desire to get even. You may fight the idea of forgiveness, feeling resistant or afraid to let go of your angry self. Perhaps you don't want to live without negative excitement; it makes you feel alive, strong, and powerful. You may believe that if you let go of your anger, you'll forget the cruel acts to which you were subjected. For instance, Meredith told her therapist, "If I let it go and forgive her, it will make what she did to me all right." Or you may prefer the idea of getting even. Evangeline said that thoughts of getting back at the guy who damaged her reputation gave her a reason to live. And Brianna promised that she would never forgive herself for the pain she caused her children during her struggle with addiction. Here, Enid shares her reluctance to forgive:

> Now in her seventies, Enid had never considered forgiveness. The word was unfamiliar to her. Yes, she could forgive the occasional insult or bad word, but not the callous and cruel treatment she had received at the hands of her mother-in-law, who passed away years ago. The anger was still there, but not to the same degree, because time did help. Now she was being told that letting go of anger, total radical forgiveness, might help her deal with a recent health crisis. Well, she was willing to try. But where should she begin? What does forgiveness feel like? Would it really change something inside of her?

Enid's questions started her on the path to experience forgiveness. As difficult as it is, it's important for you to develop the strength to detach and pull your energy back from negative situations. Imagine them as burdens you carry that you need to put down to move forward. Command yourself to use forgiveness to change direction so that you can detach from negativity, release your pain, and bring more joy into your life.

The steps you need to take to reach forgiveness are discussed in the next section.

Change—From Retribution to Forgiveness

Change is a five-stage process that moves from resistance to forgiveness (McConnaughy, Prochaska, and Velicer 1983). In this case, your goal is to forgive yourself for pain your anger caused others and forgive others for pain their anger caused you. As you go through the stages, your energy moves from a "no" current to a "yes" current.

You were in the first stage before you began reading this book. You felt helpless to change your anger, believing *this is who I am*, or you simply didn't want to change your behavior. Perhaps you liked it. When others pressured you to change, you threw a tantrum like a two-year-old, internally shouting *I won't change!*—the resistance stage. But after that, you experienced a deep longing and desire to free yourself from destructive anger, the third stage of change. At this point, you may have started to believe that you could change and anger didn't have to rule your life. The fourth stage is the "yes." Motivated, you tried the somatic exercises in this book and implemented strategies to reduce your negative thinking. The final stage of change entails expanding your consciousness. This occurs when you embrace radical forgiveness through meditation, mindfulness, visualization, and prayer.

EXERCISE: Five Stages of Change

Say each of the following statements out loud three times while stamping your feet or doing squats to connect with the ground.

1. I *can't* change my anger.

2. I *won't* change my anger.

3. I *long to* change my anger.

4. I *can* release my anger and I *will change* my behavior.

5. I *will forgive* and *let go* of anger from the past.

As you forgive yourself and others, you free yourself of the vestiges of negativity and toxic anger. Your body changes from feeling depleted, burdened, and overly sensitive to feeling alive, content, and light. By immersing yourself in the process of radical forgiveness, you get your energy back.

The Forgiveness Process

When you forgive, you disengage from the negative energy of the target of your anger, even if that person is yourself. Imagine taking a scissors and cutting the stream of negativity that runs between you and the other. Say out loud, or write in your journal, "I am no longer willing to receive your negative energy, and I forgive you." From a shamanistic perspective, you're calling your spirit back. You're breaking a negative attachment when you forgive, allowing you to return to your authentic self and experience beauty, love, and compassion without being tainted by the other's negativity.

Forgiveness is a strength; it gives you power. Forgiveness means acknowledging the pain you received or gave, but letting go of resentment, hate, jealousy, and anger. It does not mean you forget or disregard the actions. It means you make a conscious decision to move past what happened, say goodbye to that aspect of your life, and start afresh. Here's what Melody did after experiencing major sexual trauma:

Melody was raped in her dorm room by someone she thought was a friend, until he wouldn't take "no" for an answer. Traumatized, she dropped out of school. At first, she was frozen and numb, but later she felt intense rage, killing men in her dreams, and punching and stamping in her exercise class. Because she desired to return to college and go on to medical school, she didn't want this traumatic experience to hold her back. After joining a meditation class, she focused on forgiveness and was finally able to let go of her anger and rage. Now she saw her perpetrator as a marred individual whom she could forgive. In doing so she could begin the next chapter of her life.

Next is an exercise of shamanistic origin that Melody learned in her meditation group that helped her to forgive.

EXERCISE: Forgiveness and Purification

On a small piece of paper, write the name of the person you need to forgive (it can be yourself) and a few words to describe what occurred. Place a large pot in a sink, or outdoors on a windless day, fold the paper, and place it at the bottom of the pot. Close your eyes in prayer or meditation and forgive this person for the pain you experienced. Open your eyes and burn a corner of the paper to purify it by fire. Quickly, blow it out. Then run water over what is left of the paper to purify it by water. The final step it to take it outside and wave it toward the sky, purification by air, then bury it in the ground, asking the earth to purify it. Say goodbye to this painful event and to the person you have forgiven. Turn your back and walk away.

Forgiving the Perpetrator

Forgiveness can occur when you accept and understand that the person who hurt you was shaped by their life history, personality flaws, imperfections, and lack of emotional stability. Acknowledging their weaknesses and life struggles will help you let go and detach from their destructive behavior, so that you can move on. You don't have to forget what occurred; you may still carry scars, but they will no longer consume or threaten you. If it's easier to forgive someone you know, try to attain more information about the person or get to know them in more depth. Forgiveness may be a one-time event, or it may evolve over time, and you may have to deal with one horrific situation after another. Here's how Alecia described it:

> I forgave my mother in stages. At first, I didn't remember some
> of the hideous, crazy behaviors she subjected us to before she was
> medicated. She struggled with bipolar disease her whole life.
> I remember when she tried to strangle me and when she called me
> a slut. But later, more violent memories came back, like when
> she tried to push me out of the car while it was still moving.
> I dealt with each separately, doing anger release exercises for
> each situation. Much later, when I was free of bad memories,
> I was able to forgive her.

EXERCISE: Make a Forgiveness List

In your journal make two lists. List A includes the people you have already forgiven and the harm they caused you, and List B includes people you still need to forgive and what they did to cause you pain. Some people on your list may have passed away, and that is okay. Others you may never have met, such as a great grandparent, whose actions resulted in ancestral pain. Ask yourself what's the difference between the two lists. Were those on List A easier to forgive? If so, why? If you were to do a forgiveness meditation today, with whom on List B would you begin?

Forgiving Yourself

Sometimes the person you need to forgive is yourself for using your anger, purposely or accidentally, to hurt others. In some regard, your anger has also hurt you. It may have caused health issues like high blood pressure or lowered your self-esteem. To feel good about yourself and experience self-love, you need to forgive yourself.

Self-love is different from selfishness or narcissism and it is necessary for life fulfillment. You achieve it when you absolve yourself of negativity and plug into gratitude, forgiveness, and appreciation for what you've accomplished. The following exercise focuses on forgiveness and self-love.

EXERCISE: Forgiving Your True Self

Picture yourself positively, and with this image in mind, describe six of your gifts, talents, and unique qualities, then write them in your journal. Then write a second list of six life events, small or large, for which you wish to forgive yourself. For example, Adelphia wrote, "My strength is my love for science." On the forgiveness list, she wrote, "I forgive myself for refusing to take my younger brother to the playground and making him cry." This exercise helps you recognize that you have both. You can love yourself and take pride in your positive qualities and accomplishments, and you can realistically acknowledge your flaws and forgive yourself.

Forgiveness and Health

If you have health issues such as autoimmune or cardiovascular diseases, allergies, or respiratory illnesses, try introducing forgiveness into your health regimen. Because the mind and body interact, clearing your mind of negative thoughts may help your body heal. When you forgive, you let go of hurt and anger, which may result in a change in your body. Your blood pressure may lower or a rash subside. Behavioral health researchers (Goldberg 1998; LeShan 1977; Siegel and Sander 2009) find forgiveness, assertiveness, and strength factors in longevity and remission for cancer and heart disease. In forgiving, you're initiating a whole-body healing process, letting go of stress, decreasing physical arousal, and creating a healthier lifestyle.

The body scan that follows focuses on the connection between forgiveness and your body.

EXERCISE: Forgiveness Body Scan

Sit or lie in a relaxed position, close your eyes, and focus on your breathing. Imagine a small you, no bigger than a pinhead, entering your body through the top of your head and taking a trip down through your body ending at your feet. On the way, you visit parts of your body (eyes, jaw, mouth, head, neck, shoulders, upper back, lower back, chest, heart, lungs, stomach, intestines, liver, pancreas, gall bladder, uterus, genitals, arms, hands, legs, and feet) and forgive each one. Internally say, I forgive you to each body part. When you sense a softening, warmth, or energy flow in your body, then you know forgiveness has occurred. Or you may feel it as compassion or empathy. Experience the difference in your body once you've forgiven it.

Using Meditation to Forgive

Meditation is a powerful tool when it's used for forgiveness.

When you meditate, you are relaxed, clear, focused, and totally aware. Everything else drifts away. Three types of forgiveness meditations are provided here: two to forgive yourself and one to forgive others. In the first you forgive yourself for the harm your anger caused others, and in the second you forgive yourself for harm you caused yourself. The third forgives others for endangering you or causing you harm.

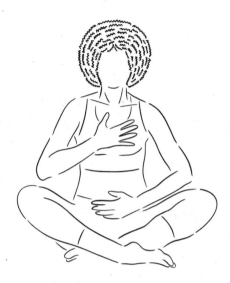

Forgiveness Through Meditation

EXERCISE 1: Harm My Anger Caused Others

Sit comfortably, eyes closed, and focus on your breath. Allow your muscles to relax. Think of those your anger harmed and ask them for forgiveness. Focus on one person at a time, saying their names. Own how you *hurt the person or caused suffering. This may have been purposeful or accidental.* Experience the pain you caused this person and apologize. "I'm sorry I hurt you by...I ask for your forgiveness." Experience this in your heart and your mind.

EXERCISE 2: Harm I Caused Myself

Sit comfortably, eyes closed, and focus on your breath. Ask your muscles to relax. Think of how you have harmed yourself with your *negative thinking, vengeful thoughts and actions, judgments, impulsive behavior, anger suppression, self-hate, and guilt* and forgive yourself. The message is *"I have hurt and harmed myself by...and I forgive myself fully with an open heart."*

EXERCISE 3: Harm Others Caused Me

Sit comfortably, eyes closed, and focus on your breath. Allow your muscles to relax. Think of those who have hurt or harmed you, one at a time. Say the name and envision how you were harmed, whether you suffered rejection, abuse, or bullying, and whether it was *purposeful or accidental. Then,* extend forgiveness to this person from your heart, saying, "I release my pain, hurt, and anger, and I offer you forgiveness."

Practice these meditations once or twice a week, making authentic forgiveness a regular part of your life. You can do them in the morning or in the evening before bed. Trust your instinct about the best time to meditate.

Forgiveness Contract

If you believe your anger has been experienced as cruel and harmful to others, you may want to write a forgiveness contract; it's a way of showing remorse and it can help you and the other release the burden of the past.

A forgiveness contract may help you and the other find peace. You may share it with the person you harmed or keep it private as a sign of your intent to seek forgiveness. If you decide to share it, consider whether it's best to do it in person or send an email or a letter. Here's a sample structure:

1. Write the name of the person you hurt with your anger.

2. Acknowledge how you caused this person pain: what you did or said.

3. Express remorse for the pain you caused, take responsibility, and apologize.

4. Commit to change, sharing that you will avoid similar situations in the future, and that you will be mindful of your words and actions.

5. Ask for forgiveness. Express understanding that it's a process, and it may take the other some time to forgive you.

6. Envision the person accepting your apology.

When you seek forgiveness, meditate, and work with your energy, you transcend your ordinary daily life and you feel as if you are part of something greater. When you ask for forgiveness, your experience is of becoming one with a greater force.

Cosmic Forgiveness: One with the Universe

Undergoing the forgiveness process is a bit unworldly. You leave darkness behind, go beyond negativity, to find the light and its healing potential. It's a transcendent, cosmic experience connecting you with something greater than yourself. You experience letting go of ego, your roles (such as wife, mother, nurse, lawyer, or mail carrier), and your day-to-day identity, needs, desires, and wants (a new car, respect, a raise). Your ego, the part that worries about what's fair, and who is right and who is wrong, recedes and your most compassionate self steps forward. In this moment you are authentic and able to experience love fully. Here's what happened to Willow:

Willow entered the room where her aunt lay dying, a woman who had once rejected her when her mother was too sick to take care of her. She sat by the bed and began to meditate, focusing on her breath. When she opened her eyes, she saw streams of beautiful, pastel-colored energy flowing around her aunt's body. It was a perfect moment. It felt like some sort of resolution had occurred. She sat peacefully at her aunt's side until the nurses told her it was time to leave. This event changed Willow's life. In the following month she joined a church. Six months later she enrolled in a pastoral studies program, and three years after that she was assigned to her first church. Meeting what appeared to her as a higher power helped Willow find her life's purpose and forgive.

Although Western psychological research lacks theories, hypotheses, and studies concerning changes in consciousness, recent brain research on samples of monks meditating supports this theory. The monks had significantly elevated gamma brain waves that fire at the highest frequency, link all parts of the brain together, and are associated with superior intelligence, compassion, happiness, and peak experiences (Adluru et al. 2020).

Forgiveness, on this higher level, involves your brain, motivation, and emotions working together as a team (Pierrakos 2014). Operating in harmony, they help you open your heart so that you can experience compassion even when you experience anger: yours or someone else's directed at you. Next is a gratitude meditation, based on reason, will, and emotion, and the role they play in forgiveness.

EXERCISE: Expressing Gratitude

Sit or lie quietly in a comfortable place. Close your eyes and breathe deeply, releasing tension from your body. Staying in the present, breathe slowly, inhaling and exhaling, and reflect on your marvelous brain, its ability to reason, think clearly, make sense out of confusion, and gather facts. Feel gratitude toward its help in the forgiveness process. Then reflect on your will and send it gratitude. The will center sits between your shoulder blades on your upper back. Breathe into it and thank it for motivating you to seek or give forgiveness. Finally, breathe into your heart, feeling any armor around it melt, as you send it gratitude for being willing to offer empathy, compassion, and forgiveness. Feel the warmth of gratitude circulate through your body. Stay peacefully relaxed for a minute or two before arising.

The Power of Prayer

Some research supports prayer's positive effects. Spiritually inclined people heal faster from illness (Zare et al. 2019). When you pray for others, called intercessory prayer, the recipients have better outcomes than those who don't receive the benefit of prayer (Byrd 1988).

Prayer, like meditation, transcends one's ordinary sense of self, bringing you in touch with a power seemingly greater than yourself. It can be used as a tool for self-reflection and self-awareness as well as help you develop a deeper understanding of what you truly value. It supports transforming toxic anger, asking for forgiveness, and giving forgiveness.

Forgiveness: Becoming One with the Universe

Forgiving involves making an offering with generosity and compassion. When you let go of resentment, you gift the person who has been receiving your negative vibes. You also gift yourself because you no longer carry this negative burden. You may even offer an opportunity for reconciliation or a second chance, although neither is necessary for forgiveness. In forgiving you also receive. When your heart opens, it reaches out tenderly toward the other. In that process, you receive back, not necessarily from the one who you are forgiving, although that can happen, but from the universe. By forgiving yourself and others, using somatic exercises including meditation, mindfulness, breathwork, and prayer, you transcend your normal, day-to-day worldly experience, let go of your ego, and your inner judge who decides who's right and who's wrong. Forgiveness gives you the gift of full body relaxation, peace, and being one with the universe and the natural world.

In Part 3 you'll have an opportunity to learn how to maintain what you've accomplished and deal with relapses if they occur. There's also a resource page to help you find outside sources to support your continued growth, meditation practices and retreats, and courses in anger management and transformation.

Part 3

FUTURE ACTIONS *and* FOLLOW-UP

CHAPTER 3

Awakening to Your Real Self

A little progress each day adds up to big results.

—Author Unknown

As she walked down the aisle to meet her wife, Benji could not believe how much she had changed. Going from an insecure person whose anger bounced off the walls if she felt the slightest hint of rejection, she had let go of this negative thinking, knowing it had to do with her mother's hostility and abandonment and not her current relationship. She was so thankful for the work she had done to release and transform her anger, knowing this wedding wouldn't be taking place if she hadn't done so.

The word "plastic" may best describe your ability to change. Just as new pathways in the brain can open for people with brain injuries, anger can be channeled along healthier routes for women who struggle with toxic anger: the impulsive expression of it or the out-of-awareness suppression of it. You're not locked into a rigid emotional system; your brain and body are both flexible and free to change. Lipton's 2005 research from the field of epigenetics shows that the DNA you inherited does not define you. Stressful situations you have been exposed to, even prior to birth, may have affected how you handle anger, but the exercises and techniques in this workbook have helped you get back on track and connect to your true identity. By freeing up energy blocked in your body, you've replaced negative, self-defeating behaviors and thoughts with positive emotions and actions. You've found new ways to connect to your anger, use it rationally, and speak your truth. Congratulations! You have accomplished a lot. The seven steps for healing toxic anger have helped you become aware of your anger and change its form.

By working holistically, mind, body, spirit, and emotion, and using somatic exercises to unblock and release your anger, you have enabled a positive energy flow. You can build relationships rather than tear them down, give empathy when under stress, problem solve, communicate respectfully, and forgive yourself and others. Your accomplishments include:

- controlling destructive venting

- expressing anger rationally rather than suppressing it

- freeing yourself from secretive, sneaky, passive-aggressive acts

- creating a better energy flow in your body

- decreasing stress in your body

- sharing angry feelings without blame or judgment

- changing negative thinking patterns to positive or neutral ones

- becoming less reactive to anger directed at you

- developing awareness of where anger lives in your body

- identifying the invisible roots that feed your anger

- grounding your anger to remain present and in reality

- employing somatic exercises and releasing techniques to create a positive energy flow

- sharing thoughts assertively and rationally

- experiencing radical forgiveness and compassion

By following the guidance in this book, your whole person has benefited. In addition to transforming your anger, you learned how to communicate it appropriately and use it for creative problem solving. You're able to quiet physiological arousal to listen to your anger and recognize its inherent wisdom. Speaking about this, Kineala said,

> *I was furious with April's teacher for suggesting holding her back, saying she's too immature for second grade. I wanted to wring her neck. After moving energy and meditating, I listened to the reason behind my anger. It wouldn't be right for April, although it might be for another child. April needed to be with her friends. It would be a blow to her self-esteem to have others move on without her. I was able to present my case rationally and we came to an agreement.*

By using your anger to solve problems and enhance relationships rather than create problems and end relationships, you are committing to a healthier lifestyle. You're aligning with a higher truth. To honor what you have accomplished, do this heart meditation, which focuses on loving yourself.

EXERCISE: Meditation to Open the Heart

Sit or lie comfortably, eyelids closed, and focus on your breathing. Experience your life force, the energy that moves through you and surrounds your body. Feel this energy in your vital organs, moving up toward your head, out into your arms and hands, and down toward your feet. Now focus on your heart and imagine it centered in your chest. See its unique shape, size, texture, scars, colors, radiance, memories, and pain. Be aware of its rhythmical beat. Sense its front, back, sides, and center. Now imagine it growing bigger so that it takes up your entire chest. Continue to breathe deeply and slowly. Be aware of any emotions that show up as your heart grows larger and welcome them. Now imagine your heart growing so big that it surrounds your entire body. You're sitting or lying within your heart. Be aware of its beauty, its wounds, its ups, and its downs.

There's a transparent door in your heart that opens and closes. If you are willing, open the door and let in love and forgiveness. After you receive the love, close the door and be aware of your feelings. Now open the door again and let in those who will support you, love you, and make you happy—pets, children, spouses or lovers, parents, relatives, ancestors, exes, friends, and colleagues, dead or alive. Invite in those who genuinely care about you. You may choose to let no one in, and that is fine too. When you have let in those you want, close the door to your heart. Envision it shrinking slowly back to its normal size. Place your palms on your chest, say thank you, and when you are ready, open your eyes and stretch. Write in your journal the thoughts and feelings that arose during this exercise.

Strategies to Sustain Freedom from Toxic Anger

To keep your momentum, consider implementing strategies to prevent relapse. Until strong habits kick in, new behaviors can falter or slip away. Some regression is normal. Change is sometimes two steps forward and one step backward. You can expect to have an occasional toxic anger episode. Accept that you are doing the best that you can and that you're a work in progress. Sustained wellness strategies will help you stay on track and manage toxic anger when stressful situations occur.

First, set aside some time to identify situations that could trigger a relapse. For example, my anger gets triggered when I feel left out. If everyone in the family is included in a group email and I'm left out, that hurts and triggers my anger.

Once you identify your high-risk situations, you can think about how you might respond, or not respond if you tend to be impulsive under stress. Then rehearse your responses by saying them aloud, or recording them, until you feel comfortable with your message and how you sound. Another option is to write your response on an index card that you can carry with you. Serena carried an index card in her wallet that read RESPOND!!! because her tendency was to overlook injuries and insults.

Then list coping behaviors that will help you decrease, transform, or present your anger in the best possible light. For example, you might cope best by taking a break from an argument to do grounding exercises or staccato breathing. Have at least three coping strategies for anger that you are prepared to use, and think about when, how, and where you will use them.

For example, Jada used her anger journal to cope. She wrote about the most recent episode, what triggered it, its intensity, and how long it lasted. She noted how it differed from her anger in the past. Here are some additional coping strategies for toxic anger. Keep a list of the strategies that work for you in your anger journal:

- Introduce more pleasure into your life, including favorite foods, concert tickets, affection, sex, and travel, to counterbalance annoyances, irritations, and general negativity.

- Create an anti-anger message to talk yourself out of responding impulsively or irrationally.

- Enumerate the benefits of controlling anger if you're prone to vent and of speaking up if you lean toward suppression.

- Write a contract committing to handle your anger in a healthy way.

- Practice relaxation, meditation, and anger release exercises three times per week to counter everyday stress and physiological arousal.

- Measure your blood pressure and keep a record, as blood pressure can indicate stress and anger.

- Have an anger buddy to discuss difficulties that arise and the best ways to handle them.

- Build a support system of several people you trust to talk with when you're upset. These can be close friends, work colleagues, or relatives. If you're introverted or lack people to call upon, think of using an online service. It will give you the opportunity to express yourself—which is a form of release.

- Be open about your need for anger management and your history with anger.

- Remind yourself of your goals and review them often. Remember why you were motivated to change your anger behavior in the first place.

- Make fewer judgments of yourself and others; commit to 50 percent less negative thinking. Catch negative thoughts before they take over your mind, especially the subliminal ones that try to sneak by. Imagine a red stoplight to stop the thought, reframe it, or just say "NO" to the thought.

- Express your anger creatively through art, knitting, poetry, short stories, blogs, letters to the editor, pottery, woodwork, and sculpture.

- Attend anger management workshops and meditation retreats.

- Don't socialize or spend time with angry, complaining, negative people. If you have no choice, disconnect your energy from theirs so they can't affect you.

- Help other people talk rationally about their anger (such as your children, spouse, parents, friends, colleagues). Teaching them will reinforce the changes you've already made.

- Set boundaries: say "no" and "I won't."

- Stay in the present moment, aware of your body, and experience your feelings without acting on them.

- Communicate your authentic feelings in as many situations as possible.

Stay in Touch with Your Authentic Self

When you lose touch with your authentic self, you have a greater tendency to regress and relapse into toxic anger. Therefore, it is important to embrace your undefended and vulnerable persona. If you find yourself behaving in any of the ways listed below, you need to take more cautions to prevent relapse.

- Driven, overworked, exhausted, and burned-out

- Helpless, victimized, abused, traumatized

- Better than others, special, right, and arrogant

- Owed, neglected, and deprived

- Less than others or rejected

- Undeserving of happiness

- Strong desire to stay separate, armored, or closed

- Too much yang, aggressive, assertive energy

- Too much yin, passive, laid-back energy

- Not enough time for relaxation, meditation, creative activities, or sitting quietly

Cindy was aware of not wanting to relapse. After completing the seven-step program, her life had never been better. Her greatest fear was shutting down again, armoring herself, and pushing newly made friends away. When she began the program, she acknowledged fearing and hating people, and not wanting to be around them. A violent, narcissistic father, who cut off a chicken's head in front of her, and a terrible junior high school rejection made her decide to close off completely.

Detached, her anger came out sideways, refusing to make eye contact, and directing hateful feelings for others toward herself, she submitted to dozens of one-night stands. During the program, Cindy began to feel at home in her body. Enjoying the sensations of flowing energy and letting go of tension, she experienced self-love for the first time. Yearning to connect with people and develop intimacy, she was in a relationship by the end of the program. Because it would be easy to shut down again, she tried to share at least one personal feeling in every conversation and she joined several online support groups.

Like Cindy, it's important for you to own your vulnerability and share feelings with family, friends, colleagues, and even strangers. Toxic anger can make you feel strong and powerful, but it lacks authenticity. When angry, empower yourself by being assertive and clear about what you are angry about and what you would like to be different in the future.

You don't have to rationalize or justify your anger. You don't need a reason for anger. Anger is normal when communicated appropriately; it's part of human biology and important for human survival. You, like every other person on the planet, will experience anger. But it doesn't have to be toxic or hurt your relationships or your health. Anger does not define you. It is a feeling that flows through you and then is gone. Toxic anger only poisons the waters because you hold on to it. You must decide how and when to share your anger. The best tool is to present your case calmly and honestly.

However, accept the inevitability of being misunderstood when you talk about anger. Even if you don't direct anger at others, they may still feel criticized. Therefore, listen to their side with empathy and set the intention to release them from needing to agree with you. Choose to salvage the relationship over being right. You may agree to disagree, simply appreciating the opportunity to have shared. Connections with others, even when confusing or chaotic, are a better option than separation and loneliness, unless those others are violent or abusive. If you have realistic expectations and recognize you can't stop anger from occurring, you will use it to enhance your relationships, find creative solutions to problems, and improve your life, even when you're on the receiving end of it.

How you receive anger that's directed at you is also important. Anger will come at you in many different forms. Behaviors from shouting to name calling to ignoring to criticizing to gaslighting to ghosting are all based on hostile and destructive emotional patterns. These actions will come from people you care about—your children, colleagues, friends, and relatives, as well as from strangers.

When anger comes toward you, you need to decide how to respond. In some cases, the person's looking for a fight and in others, they're letting off steam. Sometimes they don't like your behavior. Perhaps you recognize it's their problem and you don't have to do anything. A response other than "I hear you" or "let me think about it" is unnecessary. Don't allow yourself to become defensive and be drawn into something because someone is unhappy with your behavior unless it's meaningful, worthwhile, and you need to take a position. Then, state your case assertively.

Use the following meditation to cement your intention to maintain the changes you have made.

EXERCISE: Anger—Peace Meditation

- Find a quiet, peaceful place to sit comfortably and close your eyes. Let go of distractions.

- Breath naturally, observing your breath.

- On the in-breath, envision the word "in" and on the out-breath, the word "out," labeling each breath. Do this for a minute or two.

- If a thought passes through your mind, don't dwell on it, but let it go immediately.

- Now change the words so that on the in-breath you envision breathing in "peace" and on the out-breath you envision breathing out "anger."

- Do the exercise once daily for at least five minutes.

This meditation is a wonderful way to begin or end a day.

Soaring Ahead

Life is movement. You never want to stop growing, changing, or creating the life you want to live. You've taken a big step in rescuing yourself from the throes of toxic anger. Now you can use healthy anger, when it occurs, to move forward and enhance your life. You can step out assertively without stepping on someone else's toes.

The somatic exercises, energy techniques, and reframing of negative thoughts you learned here will help you maintain what you've accomplished and get through occasional relapses. Now you have the coping skills to deal with toxic anger and get back on track. Never forget to forgive yourself and others for human foibles and have deep gratitude for the person you are, all that you may still become, and the people you meet along the way.

Resources: More Life-Energizing Approaches

Meditation

Meditation retreats are helpful for managing toxic anger and preventing relapse as they help you relax and calm your body's natural reaction to stress. Retreat centers open and close, and schedules change, so this list can only provide a starting place for you to begin your search for a center that you find comfortable, restorative, and affordable. Please check their websites for the most up-to-date information.

Dhamma.org (Vipassana Meditation Centers)
Website: Dhamma.org

Kripalu
Website: Kripalu.org

Insight Meditation Society (IMS)
Website: Dharma.org

Mindful
Website: Mindful.org

Omega Institute
Website: EOmega.org

Plum Village (Thich Nhat Hanh's Monastic Community)
Website: Plumvillage.org

Shambhala Mountain Center
Website: Shambhala.org

Spirit Rock Meditation Center
Website: Spiritrock.org

Tara Brach—Retreats and Workshops
Website: Tarabrach.org

The Chopra Center
Website: Chopra.com

Tricycle Retreats
Website: Tricycle.org

Anger Management Courses

The following groups offer courses, trainings, and workshops for anger management and transformation.

Online Organizations

Alison.com

Coursera.com

CoursesforSuccess.com

Media Psychology Associates

DrMichaelBroder.com

Mindfulness-Based Stress Reduction (MBSR) Online.
Website: http://www.palousemindfulness.com

NICABM. Website: http://www.nicabm.com

Udemy. Website: http://www.udemy.com

Workshops and Trainings

Center for Somatic Healing.
Website: www.centerforsomatichealing.life

Core Energetics Academy. Online seminars on "Transforming Anger to Love & Compassion." Website: www.drkarynewilner.com

Exceptional Marriage. Website: www.exceptionalmarriage.com

Institute of Body Psychotherapy (Australia). Website: www.instituteofbodypsychotherapy.com

Institute of Core Energetics. Website: www.coreenergetics.org

International Institute for Core Evolution & CoreSoma. Website: www.CoreEvolution.com

Radical Aliveness. Website: www.radicalaliveness.org

Seattle School of Body-Psychotherapy. Website: https://www.bodypsychotherapyschool.com

Online Counseling

Psychology Today Directory

Search for local or national online therapists specializing in anger management.

Anger Management Workshops and Trainings

Betterhelp.com

GoodTherapy.org

References

Adluru, N., C. H. Korponay, D. L. Norton, R. I. Goldman, and R. J. Davidson. 2020. "Brainage and Regional Volumetric Analysis of a Buddhist Monk: A Longitudinal MRI Case Study." *Neurocase* 26(2): 79–90.

Ayakody, K., S. Gunadasa, and C. Hosker. 2014. "Exercise for Anxiety Disorders: Systematic Review." *British Journal of Sports Medicine* 48: 187–196.

Banafa, A., A. L. Suominen, and K. Sipila. 2023. "Association Between Cynical Hostility and Temporomandibular Pain Mediated Through Somatization and Depression: An 11-Year Follow-Up Study on Finnish Adults." *Acta Odontologica Scandinavica* 81: 79–85.

Beck, A. T. 1979. *Cognitive Therapy and the Emotional Disorders.* New York: Penguin Books.

Beck, A. T. 1999. *Prisoners of Hate: The Cognitive Basis of Anger, Hostility, and Violence.* New York: HarperCollins Publishers.

Beck, A. T., and A. Freeman. 1990. *Cognitive Therapy of Personality Disorders.* New York: Guilford Press.

Benson, H., B. R. Marzetta, and B. A. Rosner. 1974. "Decreased Blood Pressure Associated with the Regular Elicitation of the Relaxation Response: A Study of Hypertensive Subjects." In *Contemporary Problems in Cardiology, Vol. I: Stress and the Heart,* edited by R. S. Eliot. Mt. Kisco, NY: Futura.

Benson, H., and E. M. Stuart, eds. 1992. *The Wellness Book: The Comprehensive Guide to Maintaining Health and Treating Stress-Related Illness.* New York: Fireside Edition, Simon & Schuster.

Birdwhistell, R. L. 1970. *Kinesics and Context: Essays on Body Motion.* Philadelphia: University of Pennsylvania Press.

Bouchard, T. J. Jr., D. T. Lykken, M. McGue, N. L. Segal, and A. Tellegen. 1990. "Sources of Human Psychological Differences: The Minnesota Study of Twins Reared Apart." *Science* 250(4978): 223–228.

Boyle, S. W., W. Church II, and E. Byrnes. 2005. "Migraine Headaches and Anger." *Best Practices in Mental Health* 1(12): 47–58.

Brennan, B. 1988. *Hands of Light: A Guide to Healing Through the Human Energy Field*. New York: Random House.

Burns, D. 1999. *Feeling Good: The New Mood Therapy*. New York: HarperCollins Publishers.

Byrd, R. C. 1988. "Positive Therapeutic Effects of Intercessory Prayer in a Coronary Care Unit Population." *Southern Medical Journal* 81(7): 826–829.

Capon, H., M. O'Shea, S. Evans, and S. McIver. 2021. "Yoga Complements Cognitive Behavior Therapy as an Adjunct Treatment for Anxiety and Depression: Qualitative Findings from a Mixed-Methods Study." *Psychology and Psychotherapy: Theory, Research and Practice* 94(4): 1015–1035.

Chaudhury, P., and U. Banerjee. 2020. "Nature of Anger, Life Event Stress, Conflict and Defense Mechanisms Among Individuals Having Peptic Ulcer: A Comparative Study." *Psychological Studies* 65: 285–295.

Chekroud, S., R. R. Gueorguieva, A. B. Zheutlin, M. Paulus, H. M. Krumholz, J. H. Krystal, and A. M. Chekroud. 2018. "Association Between Physical Exercise and Mental Health in 1.2 Million Individuals in the USA Between 2011 and 2015: A Cross-Sectional Study." *Lancet Psychiatry* 5(9): 739–746.

Chopra, D., and M. C. Kafatos. 2018. *You Are the Universe: Discovering Your Cosmic Self and Why It Matters*. New York: Harmony Books.

Christensen, A. J., and T. W. Smith. 1993. "Cynical Hostility and Cardiovascular Reactivity During Self-Disclosure." *Psychosomatic Medicine* 55: 193–202.

Cozolino, L. 2002. *The Neuroscience of Psychotherapy: Healing the Social Brain*, 3rd ed. New York: W. W. Norton.

Craske, M. G., an D. H. Barlow. 2006. *Mastery of Your Anxiety and Worry: Workbook*, 2nd ed. Oxford: Oxford University Press.

Dubbert, P. M. 1992. "Exercise in Behavioral Medicine." *Journal of Consulting and Clinical Psychology* 60: 613–618.

Evans, I. M. 2015. *How and Why Thoughts Change: Foundations of Cognitive Therapy*. Oxford: Oxford University Press.

Everson, S. A., D. E. Goldberg, G. A. Kaplan, J. Julkunen, and J. T. Salonen. 1998. "Anger Expression and Incident Hypertension." *Psychosomatic Medicine* 60: 730–735.

Freud, S. 1960. *The Ego and the Id*. New York: W. W. Norton.

Gendlin, E. 1978. *Focusing*. New York: Bantam Dell.

Geronimus, A. T. 2023. *Weathering: The Extraordinary Stress of Ordinary Life in an Unjust Society*. New York: Little, Brown Spark.

Goldberg, B. 1998. *Heart Disease, Stroke, & High Blood Pressure: Heart Problems Can Be Prevented and Reversed Using Clinically Proven Alternative Therapies*. Tiburon, CA: Future Medicine Publishing.

Goldfried, M. R., and D. Sobocinski. 1975. "Effect of Irrational Beliefs on Emotional Arousal." *Journal of Consulting and Clinical Psychology* 43: 503–510.

Goleman, D., and J. Gurin, eds. 1993. *Mind Body Medicine: How to Use Your Mind for Better Health*. Yonkers, NY: Consumer Reports Books.

Gottman, J. M., and R. W. Levenson. 2000. "The Timing of Divorce: Predicting When a Couple Will Divorce Over a 14-Year Period." *Journal of Marriage and the Family* 62: 737–745.

Guidi, J., M. Lucente, N. Sonino, and A. F. Giovanni. 2021. "Allostatic Load and Its Impact on Health: A Systematic Review." *Psychotherapy and Psychosomatics* 90(1): 11–27.

Hahn, T. N. 1975. *The Miracle of Mindfulness: An Introduction to the Practice of Meditation*. Boston: Beacon Press.

Harburg, E., M. Julius, N. Kaciroti, and L. Bleiberman. 2003. "Expressive/Suppressive Anger-Coping Responses, Gender, and Types of Mortality: A 17-Year Follow-Up (Tecumseh, Michigan, 1971–1988)." *Psychosomatic Medicine* 65(4): 588–597.

Huddleston, J. J. 1992. "Living with Heart Disease and Diabetes: Exercise Can Help." In *The Wellness Book: The Comprehensive Guide to Maintaining Health and Treating Stress-Related Illness*, edited by H. Benson and E. M. Stuart, 400–420. New York: Fireside Edition, Simon & Schuster.

Jacob, R. G., A. P. Shapiro, P. O'Hara, S. Portser, A. Kruger, C. Gatsonis, et al. 1992. "Relaxation Therapy for Hypertension: Setting-Specific Effects." *Psychosomatic Medicine* 54: 87–101.

Jacobson, E. 1938. *Progressive Relaxation*. Chicago: University of Chicago Press.

Jacobson, E. 1976. "Who Can Be Relaxed?" In *Relax: How You Can Feel Better, Reduce Stress and Overcome Tension*, edited by J. White and J. Fadiman. New York: Confucian Press.

Julkunen, J., U. Idanpaan-Heikkila, and T. Saarinen. 1993. "Components of Type A Behavior and the First-Year Prognosis of a Myocardial Infarction." *Journal of Psychosomatic Research* 37(1): 1–18.

Kabat-Zinn, J. 2013. *Full Catastrophe Living (Revised Edition): Using the Wisdom of Your Body and Mind to Face Stress, Pain, and Illness.* New York: Bantam Books.

Karp, H. 2015. *The Happiest Baby on the Block; Fully Revised and Updated Second Edition: The New Way to Calm Crying and Help Your Newborn Baby Sleep Longer.* New York: Bantam Books.

Knox, S. S., and D. Follmann. 1993. "Gender Difference in the Psychosocial Variance of Framingham and Bortner Type A Measures." *Journal of Psychosomatic Research* 37(7): 709–716.

Lahad, A., S. R. Heckbert, T. D. Koepsell, B. M. Psaty, and D. L. Patrick. 1997. "Hostility, Aggression and the Risk of Nonfatal Myocardial Infarction in Postmenopausal Women." *Journal of Psychosomatic Research* 43(2): 183–195.

Lai, R. Y., and W. Linden. 1992. "Gender, Anger Expression Style, and Opportunity for Anger Release Determine Cardiovascular Reaction to and Recovery from Anger Provocation." *Psychosomatic Medicine* 54: 297–310.

Lange, A. 2011. "Prenatal Maternal Stress and Developing Fetus and Infant: A Review of Animal Models as Restated to Human Research." *Journal of Infant, Child, and Adolescent Psychotherapy* 10(2–3): 326–340.

Lawler, K. A., T. L. Harralson, C. A. Armstead, and L. A. Schmied. 1993. "Gender and Cardiovascular Responses: What Is the Role of Hostility?" *Journal of Psychosomatic Research* 37(6): 603–613.

Lawler, K. A., Z. C. Wilcox, and S. F. Anderson. 1995. "Gender Differences in Patterns of Dynamic Cardiovascular Regulation." *Psychosomatic Medicine* 57: 357–365.

Lehrer, P. 2006. "Anger, Stress, Dysregulation Produces Wear and Tear on the Lung." *Thorax* 61(10): 833–834.

LeShan, L. 1977. *You Can Fight for Your Life: Emotional Factors in the Causation of Cancer.* New York: Rowman and Littlefield.

Linkins, R. W., and G. W. Comstock. 1990. "Depressed Mood and Development of Cancer." *American Journal of Epidemiology* 132: 962–972.

Lipton, H. B. 2005. *The Biology of Belief: Unleashing the Power of Consciousness, Matter, and Miracles.* Carlsbad, CA: Hay House.

Lowen, A. 1958. *The Language of the Body.* Springfield, OH: Collier Books.

Lowen, A., and L. Lowen. 1977. *The Way to Vibrant Health: A Manual of Bioenergetic Exercises.* New York: Harper & Row Publishers.

Maas, A. H., and Y. E. Appelman. 2010. "Gender Differences in Coronary Heart Disease." *Netherlands Heart Journal* 18(12): 598–602.

MacDougall, J. M., T. M. Dembroski, J. E. Dimsdale, and T. P. Hackett. 1985. "Components of Type A, Hostility, and Anger-In: Further Relationships to Angiographic Findings." *Health Psychology* 4(2): 37–152.

Mahler, M., F. Pine, and A. Bergman. 2000. *Psychological Birth of the Human Infant: Symbiosis and Individuation*. New York: Basic Books.

Malarkey, W. B., J. K. Kiecolt-Glaser, D. Pearl, and R. Glaser. 1994. "Hostile Behavior During Marital Conflict Alters Pituitary and Adrenal Hormones." *Psychosomatic Medicine* 56: 41–51.

Marmot, M., and E. Brunner. 2005. "Cohort Profile: The Whitehall II Study." *International Journal of Epidemiology* 34(2): 251–256.

Martin, R., E. E. I. Gordon, and P. Lounsbury. 1998. "Gender Disparities in the Attribution of Cardiac-Related Symptoms: Contribution of Commonsense Models of Illness." *Health Psychology* 17(4): 346–357.

Maté, G., and D. Maté. 2022. *The Myth of Normal: Trauma, Illness, & Healing in a Toxic Culture*. New York: Avery.

McConnaughy, E., J. Prochaska, and W. Velicer. 1983. "Stages of Change in Psychotherapy: Measurement and Sample Profiles." *Psychotherapy: Theory, Research & Practice* 20(3): 368–375.

McKay, M., P. D. Rogers, and J. McKay. 2003. *When Anger Hurts: Quieting the Storm Within*, 2nd ed. Oakland, CA: New Harbinger Publications.

Meany, M. 2018. "Prenatal Maternal Depressive Symptoms as an Issue for Population Health." *American Journal of Psychiatry* 175(11): 1084–1093.

Morris, T., S. Greer, K. W. Pettingale, and M. Watson. 1981. "Patterns of Expression of Anger and Their Psychological Correlates in Women with Breast Cancer." *Journal of Psychosomatic Research* 25(2): 111–117.

Myss, C. 1996. *Anatomy of the Spirit: The Seven Stages of Power and Healing*. New York: Harmony Books, Penguin Random House.

Nabb, J. 1999. *Core Energetic Concepts for Grounding*. Santa Fe, NM: Southwest Center for Core Energetics.

Office on Women's Health, US Department of Health and Human Services (OWH). 2023. "Diseases and Conditions." OWH. https://www.womens health.gov/heart-disease-and-stroke/heart-disease.

Pennebaker, J. W., J. K. Kiecolt-Glaser, and S. L. Glaser. 2003. "Emotional and Physical Health Benefits of Expressive Writing." *Advances in Psychosomatic Medicine* 13(2): 127–129.

Pierrakos, E. 1996. *Pathwork Lecture No. 43: Three Basic Personality Types: Reason, Will, Emotion.* Madison, VA: International Pathwork Foundation. https://pathwork.org/lecture-categories/pathwork-lectures-1996-ed.

Pierrakos, E., and D. Thesenga. 1993. *Fear No Evil: The Pathwork Method of Transforming the Lower Self.* Charlottesville, VA: Pathwork Press.

Pierrakos, J. C. 1974. *The Case of the Broken Heart.* Pamphlet. New York: Institute for the New Age of Man.

Pierrakos, J. C. 1987. *Core Energetics: Developing the Capacity to Love and Heal.* Mendocino, CA: LifeRhythm Publications.

Pierrakos, J. C. 1995. *Energy Types.* Personal communication, May 21. New York: Institute of Core Energetics.

Pierrakos, J. C. 1997. *Eros, Love & Sexuality: The Forces That Unify Man and Woman.* Mendocino, CA: LifeRhythm Publications.

Powell, L. H., L. A. Shaker, B. A. Jones, L. V. Vaccarino, C. E. Thoresen, and J. R. Pattillo. 1993. "Psychosocial Predictors of Mortality in 83 Women with Premature Acute Myocardial Infarction." *Psychosomatic Medicine* 55: 426–433.

Reich, W. 1972. *Character Analysis,* 3rd ed. New York: Touchstone Books.

Rein, G., M. Atkinson, and R. McCraty. 1995. "The Physiological Effects of Compassion and Anger." *Journal of Advancement in Medicine* 8(2): 87–105.

Rimes, K. A., J. Ashcroft, L. Bryan, and T. Chalder. 2016. "Emotional Suppression in Chronic Fatigue Syndrome: Experimental Study." *Health Psychology* 35(9): 979–986.

Rodriguez, J. C. F. 2012. "The Experience and Expression of Anger and Anxiety in Bronchial Asthma Patients." *Anuario de Psicologia* 42(2): 213–225.

Sarieddine, S. 2018. "Learning Spiritual Behaviors as a Means to Reverse Harmful Epigenetic Changes Resulting from Domestic Violence." *CPQ Neurology and Psychology* 1: 1–11.

Selye, H. 1978. *The Stress of Life,* rev. ed. New York: McGraw Hill.

Shapiro, F., and M. S. Forrest. 2016. *EMDR: The Breakthrough Therapy for Overcoming Anxiety, Stress, and Trauma.* New York: Basic Books.

Siegel, B., and J. Sander. 2009. *Faith, Hope and Healing: Inspiring Lessons Learned from People Living with Cancer.* New York: John Wiley & Sons.

Simonton, C. O., and S. M. Simonton. 1980. *Getting Well Again: The Bestselling Classic About the Simontons' Revolutionary Lifesaving Self-Awareness Techniques.* New York: Bantam Books.

Singh, B., T. Olds, R. Curtis, R. D. Dumuid, R. Vigara, A. Watson, et al. 2023. "Effectiveness of Physical Activity Interventions for Improving Depression, Anxiety and Distress: An Overview of Systematic Reviews." *British Journal of Sports Medicine* 57: 1203–1209.

Smyth, J. M., M. J. Zawadzki, A. M. Santuzzi, and K. B. Filipkowski. 2014. "Examining the Effects of Perceived Social Support on Momentary Mood and Symptom Reports in Asthma and Arthritis Patients." *Psychology & Health* 29: 813–831.

Spielberger, C. D., G. Jacobs, S. Russell, and R. S. Crane. 1983. "Assessment of Anger: The State-Trait Anger Scale." In *Advances in Personality Assessment, Vol. 2*, edited by J. D. Butcher and C. D. Spielberger. Hillsdale, NJ: Erlbaum.

Stern, D. N. 1990. *Diary of a Baby*. New York: Basic Books.

Suarez, E. C., C. M. Kuhn, S. M. Schanberg, R. B. Williams Jr., and E. A. Zimmermann. 1998. "Neuroendocrine, Cardiovascular, and Emotional Responses of Hostile Men: The Role of Interpersonal Challenge." *Psychosomatic Medicine* 60: 78–88.

Suinn, R. M. 2001. "The Terrible Twos—Anger and Anxiety: Hazardous to Your Health (Presidential Address)." *American Psychologist* 56(1): 27–36.

Truglia, E., E. Mannucci, S. Lassi, C. M. Rotella, C. Faravelli, and V. Ricca. 2006. "Aggressiveness, Anger and Eating Disorders: A Review." *Psychopathology* 39(2): 55–68.

Turk, D., D. Meichenbaum, and M. Genest. 1983. *Pain and Behavioral Medicine: A Cognitive-Behavioral Perspective*. New York: Guilford Press.

Vögele, C., A. Jarvis, and K. Cheeseman. 1997. "Anger Suppression, Reactivity, and Hypertension Risk: Gender Makes a Difference." *Annals of Behavioral Medicine* 19: 61–69.

Whitehead, W. E. 1992. "Behavioral Approaches to Gastrointestinal Disorders." *Journal of Consulting and Clinical Psychology* 60(4): 605–614.

Wilner, K. B. 1999. "Core Energetics: Action Methods for Bodily Energy and Consciousness." In *Beyond Talk Therapy: Using Movement and Expressive Techniques in Clinical Practice*, edited by D. J. Wiener, 183–204. Washington, DC: American Psychological Association.

Wilner, K. B. 2004. *An Investigation of Anger Management Techniques for Hypertension Patients*. Philadelphia: Philadelphia College of Osteopathic Medicine.

Wilner, K. B. 2012. Class Discussion, Department of Holistic Counseling, Graduate Students in Body Orientation Course. Newport, RI: Salve Regina University.

Wilner, K. B. 2020. "The Wounding Womb: Healing Prenatal Trauma." *International Body Psychotherapy Journal: The Art and Science of Somatic Praxis* 19(2): 55–62.

Wilner, K. B., and S. Black. 2009. *Techniques Used by John C. Pierrakos, MD.* Newtown, CT: The Institute of Core Energetics.

Wolman, B. B. 1988. *Psychosomatic Disorders*. New York: Plenum Publishing.

Young, D. R. 1994. "Can Cardiovascular Fitness Moderate the Negative Effects of Stress on Coronary Artery Disease Risk Factors?" *Journal of Psychosomatic Research* 38(5): 451–459.

Young, L. D. 1992. "Psychological Factors in Rheumatoid Arthritis." *Journal of Consulting and Clinical Psychology* 60(4): 619–627.

Zare, A., N. J. Bahia, F. Eidy, N. Adib, and F. Sedge. 2019. "The Relationship Between Spiritual Well-Being, Mental Health, and Quality of Life in Cancer Patients Receiving Chemotherapy." *Journal of Family Medicine and Primary Care* 8(5): 1701–1705.

Zonderman, A. B., P. T. Costa, and R. R. McCrae. 1989. "Depression as a Risk for Cancer Morbidity and Mortality in a Nationally Representative Sample." *Journal of the American Medical Association* 269(9): 1191–1195.

Zschucke, E., K. Gaudlitz, and A. Ströhle. 2013. "Exercise and Activity in Mental Disorders: Clinical and Experimental Evidence." *Journal of Preventive Medicine and Public Health* 46: S12–S21.

Zweig, C., and J. Abrams, eds. 1991. *Meeting the Shadow: The Hidden Power of the Dark Side of Human Nature*. New York: Penguin Group.

Karyne B. Wilner, PsyD, is a licensed psychologist with a private practice in Newport, RI. She currently directs the Core Energetics Academy in Bethel, CT; and was formerly assistant director of the International Institute for Core Energetics, senior director of the Brazilian Institute, and associate director in Australia. She has traveled widely giving lectures, workshops, and seminars, and has written numerous journal articles about somatic therapy and psychology. In addition to her therapist training programs, she directed Drexel University's Counseling Center in Philadelphia, PA; and she taught master's level holistic counseling courses at Salve Regina University in Newport, RI, from 2010 through 2022. Her joy lies in helping people become more authentic and lead richer, fuller lives.

Foreword writer **Teressa Moore Griffin** is an organization development consultant, executive coach, author, radio personality, online media thought leader, and speaker. Teressa has worked with domestic and international companies, supporting the growth and success of current and emerging C-level executives since 1987. A self-awareness and personal growth expert, Teressa skillfully helps clients uncover their strengths, clarify their goals, and eliminate beliefs that limit their success and satisfaction.

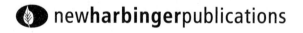

MORE BOOKS from
NEW HARBINGER PUBLICATIONS

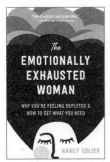
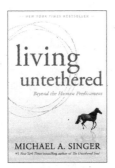
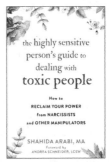
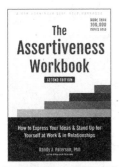
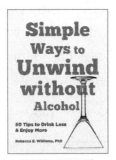
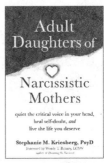

Did you know there are **free tools** you can download for this book?

Free tools are things like **worksheets, guided meditation exercises**, and **more** that will help you get the most out of your book.

You can download free tools for this book— whether you bought or borrowed it, in any format, from any source—from the New Harbinger website. All you need is a NewHarbinger.com account. Just use the URL provided in this book to view the free tools that are available for it. Then, click on the "download" button for the free tool you want, and follow the prompts that appear to log in to your NewHarbinger.com account and download the material.

You can also save the free tools for this book to your **Free Tools Library** so you can access them again anytime, just by logging in to your account! Just look for this button on the book's free tools page.

+ Save this to my free tools library

If you need help accessing or downloading free tools, visit **newharbinger.com/faq** or contact us at **customerservice@newharbinger.com**.